# LaStone
# THERAPY

*Other Books by Jane Scrivner*

Detox Yourself
Detox Your Mind
Detox Your Life
The Little Book of Detox
Total Detox
The Quick-Fix Hangover Detox
Stay Young Detox
Jane Scrivner's Water Detox
48 Hour Detox

# LaStone
# THERAPY

## THE AMAZING NEW FORM OF
## HEALING BODYWORK THAT WILL
## TRANSFORM YOUR HEALTH

# JANE SCRIVNER

PIATKUS

*For Mary for introducing me to the stones and for Rita so she can say someone wrote a book that was dedicated to her!*

## ⠸ Visit the Piatkus website!

· · · · · · · · · · · · · · · · · · · · · · · · · · · · · · · · · ·

Piatkus publishes a wide range of best-selling fiction and non-fiction, including books on health, mind, body and spirit, sex, self-help, cookery, biography and the paranormal.

*If you want to:*
- read descriptions of our popular titles
- buy our books over the Internet
- take advantage of our special offers
- enter our monthly competition
- learn more about your favourite Piatkus authors

**VISIT OUR WEBSITE AT: www.piatkus.co.uk**

Copyright © 2003 by Jane Scrivner

First published in 2003 by
Judy Piatkus (Publishers) Limited
5 Windmill Street
London WIT 2JA
e-mail: info@piatkus.co.uk

ISBN 0 7499 2333 4

Edited by Krystyna Mayer
Text design by Paul Saunders

Typeset by Action Publishing Technology, Gloucester
Printed and bound in Wales by
Cambrian Printers, Aberystwyth

# Contents

# Introduction

LASTONE THERAPY CHANGES LIVES. It transformed Mary Nelson's, and it changed mine when it was least expected. We watch with excitement how it changes the life of every therapist we instruct, and every person that receives a treatment from the growing number of LaStone therapists around the world. Some changes are small and some are huge, but there is no doubt that LaStone Therapy is a catalyst for change.

This book is not meant to be a manual on how to do a treatment but more a guide to show you just how phenomenally effective and deeply penetrating this treatment can be. Simply by reading the book you will feel rested and more grounded. You will have learnt a lot about how nature can effect a change within us if we just know a little more about it and respect it a lot more. You may even decide to book in for a treatment and experience everything that you have read about. However, the book is not meant to be a technical step-by-step breakdown of a treatment; it is more an invitation to experience something new, by either reading or feeling.

LaStone Therapy changes you on a physical, emotional and spiritual level. LaStone Therapy balances. If you are sluggish it invigorates; if you are unhealthy it helps your body to become healthy or at least puts it in a position to fight illness more efficiently. If your immune system is weak it will be boosted, and if you are feeling down the therapy will bring you back up.

Wherever your own personal, perfect balance is, LaStone will be able to show you the way there. It may blow you out of the water on the way and give you a rollercoaster of feelings and sensations, but by the end of the treatment you will reach your own place of total balance.

The therapy makes you feel quite amazing, and it takes you through feelings you didn't know you could feel good about. A true LaStone Therapy treatment is a challenge to the body, a rest for the mind and a journey for the spirit. Much of a LaStone treatment can be explained scientifically, but much is left to the individual and the universe. I cannot explain step by step exactly what happens during a treatment as it is different for everyone, but I can go some way to describing the responses people have had.

There is nothing new in LaStone Therapy. Stones have been around as long as the Earth has; hot and cold have been used in alternation in treatments for ages; the stones used are millions of years old; everyone knows about massage. What is new and totally unique is the delivery of the LaStone treatment. LaStone combines massage, thermotherapy, energy work and healing work, and it is all delivered through the very 'alive' gifts of Mother Earth – the stones.

LaStone Therapy may be one of the newest treatments available, but it is grounded in some of the oldest, most valuable, and most tried and tested therapies known to us. It is at once the newest, most advanced natural treatment available, and the oldest, most valuable and profound therapy you can have. To learn from the stones is to study under the oldest and wisest teachers.

LaStone Therapy is the ultimate dichotomy, the furthest of extremes: hot and cold, basalt and marble, Sun and Moon, male and female, yin and yang, black and white, relaxing and invigorating, sedating and euphoric, active and passive, vasodilation and vasoconstriction, Mother Earth and Father Sky.

Stones have been used in ceremony and treatments that are as old as the Incas, the Shang Dynasty in China of around 1500 BC and the Egyptian Pyramids. Native Americans have respected the Stone Clan People (as the special stones are known to them) since their time began. Using them for worship, guidance and healing, they know them and respect them as the Ancient Ones.

The alternate application of hot and cold – which is known as thermotherapy – was documented as early as the 18th century, but it is believed that the use of hot and cold bathing was an integral part of ancient Greek Hippocratic beliefs (Hippocrates died c. 430 BC).

Massage too can be traced back to Greek and Roman physicians. Hippocrates wrote: 'The physician must be experienced in many things, but assuredly in rubbing ... for rubbing can bind a joint that is too loose, and loosen a joint that is too rigid'. Hopefully we have moved on a little from basic 'rubbing', but the principles are all there.

Energy and healing work is an integral part of many ancient cultures. The Chinese have Chi or Qi, the Japanese Ki, Indians work with Prana and Reiki practitioners use the influence of the Universal Life Force. We have meridians, auric fields and chakras. We work with crystals and vibrations; we use guides and spirits, and we can work with much, much more. Almost every indigenous tribe, culture and group has a belief structure that can be incorporated into the treatment. The respect for the individual is never compromised – simply balanced and healed.

LaStone Therapy is the ultimate treatment. It is often known as the 'Last One Therapy', or the last word in therapy. LaStone Therapy is called a therapy because it is many things. It can be any therapy that you know but delivered by way of a stone – a hot and/or cold stone.

It can be aromatherapy, deep-tissue massage, remedial massage, reflexology, healing, shiatsu massage, acupressure, Chinese medicine, facials, manicures, pedicures, relaxation therapy and any other therapy. The stones know no boundaries, only the imagination of the therapist.

As with all great things, LaStone Therapy has been copied or followed. There are now many, many versions around the world. Some are more successful than others, but they all respect the power, energy and mystery of the stones.

In this book we explore the theories, origins and ideas that have combined to become LaStone Therapy. We look at the experience and the results of the stones' teaching, and the way in which the originator, Mary Nelson, has developed this treatment to put it out into the world.

We leave 'no stone unturned'. We look at how people are drawn to the stones – just as you were drawn to this book. Maybe your home contains pieces of driftwood, pebbles on window ledges, bits of rock picked up for no known reason, except that you just wanted to hold them and move them around in your hands.

We look at the technology and the chemical changes manifested in the body after or during a treatment. We look at the evidence to support the fact that LaStone Therapy is probably the most profound complementary therapy treatment available today.

CHAPTER ONE

# What is LaStone Therapy?

THERE ARE MANY, MANY FACETS to LaStone Therapy, and each is covered in detail in this book. Through a combination of detailed factual information, personal letters from Mary Nelson herself and testimonials from clients and therapists, you should be able to get a clear picture of this amazing therapy. Just see how long it takes before you want to book yourself in for a treatment.

LaStone Therapy was introduced in 1993 by Mary Nelson of Tucson, Arizona in the United States. At the time Mary was a massage therapist who wanted to find a way to be able to work more deeply without causing further damage to her own joints and muscles. She is also very spiritual, and it was this combination that led her to the stones. Her Native American spirit guide channelled to her the LaStone Therapy treatment in its entirety, and also gave it the name that is still used today.

LaStone Therapy uses heated and frozen stones to deliver the deeply therapeutic, relaxing, grounding, deep-tissue and cleansing treatment. The principles of thermotherapy, geothermotherapy, deep-tissue manipulation, auric field work, chakra response and spirituality are all used in perfect combination. The name LaStone Therapy can therefore be reworked to read 'Last One Therapy' – the last word in therapy.

LaStone is a journey that can begin with the energy work and spiritual awakenings that are experienced with the aura and placement sequences – suited to the healing and more holistic client and therapist. Alternatively, it can be approached with a view to the chemical and physical change of the body and structures that come about as a result of thermotherapy – ideally suited to the sports and remedial therapist and the client wanting deeper work. Whatever your current philosophy, and whether you are a therapist or client, there is a level of LaStone Therapy that anyone can get to grips with.

It is actually very hard to sum up what LaStone Therapy is, as it can be so many things. This is Mary Nelson's response to that very question.

'What is LaStone Therapy?' is a question I get asked all the time. Clinically it is the application of thermotherapy, using heated stones alternating with extremely cold stones for deep, penetrating bodywork. Using different temperatures, whether hot or cold, on the body to bring about a certain reaction has been done for aeons. Adjusting temperatures in bodywork to aid clients in healing has always been beneficial. LaStone Therapy will show you a way to use these different temperatures, in conjunction with Mother Earth and the Stone Clan People, to bring about balance and healing in your clients. Bring Mother Earth and the stones' energies into the treatment and let them do the walking along the muscles, allowing clients to reconnect with the inner strength of Mother Earth.

Remember what it was like as a child to lie upon the Earth and feel as though nothing in the world was wrong? People search far and wide for that sense of well-being, We have forgotten where to find it. In the fast-paced society we live in, we rarely take time to go outdoors and reconnect with the world of nature. It is too convenient to go to the gym, and some of us even have workout equipment at home. We miss the true meaning of why we go outside at all, not remembering that we need the connection to Mother Earth as much as we need to exercise. This is why LaStone Therapy is so popular: the energies of the stones remind us of our connection with Mother Earth, allowing us to feel cradled and protected.

A contemporary approach to alternating temperatures in massage, LaStone Therapy is a multifaceted technique designed to benefit client and therapist at once. The therapeutic potential of this treatment goes beyond ordinary massage. The physiological benefits of alternating heat and cold to alleviate strains to limbs have long been scientifically and medically proven.

LaStone Therapy capitalises on these traditional practices with a current approach. Basalt and marble stones are the medium, and hot and cold temperatures are the message. These 'vascular gymnastics' of the circulatory system assist the body in self-healing. LaStone Therapy administers this treatment with unerring elegance.

Therapists discover that the stress and strain to their hands, wrists and arms are virtually eliminated with this technique. The stones and thermal variation do all the heavy work for them. They are able to work more efficiently for longer periods of time.

Those who take this training develop more reverence for their daily work and rituals, because respect and appreciation grow naturally from this fertile learning experience.

LaStone Therapy produces alternately sedative and energising responses. Clients love the potent recharge they receive from the treatment. LaStone Therapy goes beyond the physical experience of typical massage, and enters deeper dimensions of relaxation, health and well-being, creating a positive approach to 'Body-Mind-Spirit' philosophy.

Not only is LaStone Therapy an advancement in therapeutic massage; it is also an absolute solution to the strain and injuries to wrists and thumbs that massage therapists experience daily.

Utilising LaStone Therapy eliminates strain to the thumbs, and helps to maintain healthy wrists by preventing hyper-flexion and hyper-extension. Let the stones do the heavy work for you. Give your thumbs and wrists a long-deserved rest. Mastering the art of LaStone Therapy will not only increase your clientele; it will also add many years to your career as a massage therapist.

LaStone Therapy is the means by which I am able to aid clients to balance their emotional, mental, physical and spiritual energies, often unlocking blocked memories, and facilitating remembrance of where they came from and who they are in this spiritual universe.

## The Treatment

As a client, the treatment will last for around an hour and fifteen minutes, depending on your current state of health. During this period your entire body is worked for the whole time. In normal massage therapy you have each limb worked for a short period of time, so that by the end of the treatment you have had your whole body worked. The legs get five minutes, the face ten and so on. No wonder the after-effects don't last very long – having your leg massaged for ten minutes each month is hardly going to have a huge effect.

LaStone works all of you, on every level, for the entire duration of the treatment – if it is ten minutes long you get the whole body worked for ten minutes; if it is over an hour long the whole body is constantly worked for over an hour, the whole time. Every part of the body is treated for every minute of the treatment, and the residual effect of the energy work and alternating temperature results in the treatment lasting for many days. Stones are constantly present, which means that temperature is constantly present. Energetic exchange is constantly happening, which means that the treatment is constant in every way.

During the treatment the therapist will place stones for you to lie on. Each stone is placed to stimulate or sedate the central nervous system, to work the muscles, to increase the blood supply and to comfort you. The therapist will place stones on you and will hold stones throughout the treatment in their hands, working them deep into the muscles; it is as if they had miraculously transformed the stones into warm and firm, turbo-charged massage tools. The placing of the stones is not random: each stone and its temperature is specifically chosen for the work the stone is required to do. Some stones are worked and removed, and some are worked and tucked in for a prolonged effect.

If you are able to have a treatment from one of the few 'advanced' or Master LaStone therapists, you will also be able to feel the effect of frozen stones as they work efficiently to instantly remove pain and tension. Even if you don't like the idea of cold stones being used, you will soon learn that they are every bit as balancing, relaxing and cleansing as the heated stones. I promise you!

To start the treatment, you will receive energy work to enable you to receive the treatment at its best. It is this work and the alternating temperatures that set LaStone apart from the more recent 'stone' treatments on the market. The combination of the energy work and the chemical response within the body during a LaStone treatment demonstrates the flexibility and the balance of the treatment. It is at once deep and remedial, as well as healing, releasing and refreshing.

## The Stones

There is nothing new about the use of stones for healing. The Chinese, Russians, Japanese, Hawaiian Kahunas, Mayan Indians and Mapuche healers of Chile have all used stones for ritual and healing over thousands of years. We have Stonehenge and stone circles, and we do crystal work to show that stones have been used through the ages for their healing properties and powers.

Just think about how many pebbles you have collected because they make you smile and feel good, even just by looking at them on the window ledge. Their qualities are very interesting. LaStone Therapy uses volcanic basalt and marble for the treatment. Both types of stone are ideally suited to heating and cooling respectively. It is this combination that yet again promotes the balance of the treatment, the yin and yang, the male and female, the black and white, the dark and night, the Sun and Moon, and the receiving and releasing.

Not only do the stones deliver the temperature; they also pass on their own personal energy. The stones come from the Earth and they are hundreds of thousands of years old. They have the resonance of the Earth and this passes to the client, energising or relaxing them. The heated stones are basalt and they are naturally formed pebbles, but the marble is hand carved and shaped to be able to do the optimum massage. The stones are used in sets and pairs in order to make the strokes feel just as balanced and smooth as the therapist's hands are.

The further beauty of the treatment is that it can extend the life of a therapist by many years. Most practitoners of bodywork suffer at one time or another from injury, strained muscles and aching joints; indeed, they often wish they, rather than their clients, could be lying on the table! LaStone takes the pressure off the joints, allows the therapist to work deeply without tiredness and actually gives the therapist a treatment at the same time as the client, because the therapist receives the temperature from the stones throughout the treatment.

In LaStone Therapy the stones are the workers, while the therapist becomes the apprentice or assistant, and is almost humbled in the presence of such knowledgeable tools. The stones seem to be naturally programmed to find the areas of pain or discomfort. We are constantly learning from the profound effects they can have. We are also constantly amazed at how the stones enable us to use our intuition to apply a stone heated to the right temperature to the right part of the body in exactly the right way.

When carrying out a LaStone treatment, one of the most common reactions from the client is surprise that the therapist seemed to know the very spot that was causing the discomfort, that every part of the client's body was addressed in the exact way it was crying out for, and that the stones were placed in the perfect positions. The client is lost for words as to how 'tailored to suit' the treatment seems to be.

Once you have worked with the stones you don't need to think too much. Very soon a stone will tell you exactly where it needs to be, for how long and at what temperature, and as soon as it needs to change it just lets you know.

There is nothing suprising about the stones once you understand that their work is perfect, and their knowledge is deep. They do, after all, have many thousands of years of learning – we just need to learn to trust them and to tap in to their wisdom.

## Thermotherapy

The use of hot stones is what intrigues clients – the feeling of being warm and relaxed appeals to everyone. The idea of the frozen stones is not always as appealing, but it is the cold that does the deepest work. The cold is extremely effective and if the therapist applies it correctly and sympathetically, the client won't actually notice the temperature; they will just feel the difference between before and after the treatment.

Too much heat can be damaging, just as too much cold can be unpleasant and chilling. A perfect balance is required: the heat relaxes and the cold invigorates, the heat pulls blood and the cold pushes it, the heat increases and the cold decreases. The balanced application of thermotherapy is one of the most effective aspects of the treatment.

We don't actually go a long way to changing the body temperature. What we do is to stimulate the body and the nervous system sufficiently to provoke a reaction and internal responses as if we had. The use of alternating temperatures is what sets LaStone apart. We truly understand the importance of balance – not too hot and not too cold, just perfect.

## The Clients' Responses

It is all very well having an amazingly effective treatment on paper, but what do people actually think after having a treatment?

Many people describe the LaStone treatment as being very nurturing and extremely relaxing. They say it is the deepest treatment they have ever experienced. This means deep on the physical level, involving working the muscles to bring the individual to full flexibility and remove pain derived from a constant state of tension and stress. It also means deep as in deep relaxation – to a level they have probably never experienced and certainly never so quickly. Within moments of being rolled onto the stones placed perfectly on either side of the spine, clients begin to relax in a way they never have before.

Deep treatment is also experienced on some other plane, on some level that clients are not sure about but where they feel safe and can feel healthy and balanced once again. There is a quintessence with LaStone that you cannot put your finger on, although you do know for sure that something has happened to you – you just don't quite know what.

The stones act like lots of little hot-water bottles 'tucked in' and left to send you off to sleep. At first it can feel a little strange, but as soon as the stones melt the muscles the feeling is of deep relaxation, grounding and centring. This feeling of deep relaxation is combined with deep-tissue manipulation that is less painful than normal massage therapy as the muscles have been thoroughly warmed – again, the stones and the temperature do the work, not the therapist.

LaStone is an all-round treatment, suited to those looking for stress release, relaxation and balancing, or to those needing a thorough workout on their body to be able to move away from injury and into total fitness.

CHAPTER TWO

The Origins of
LaStone Therapy

I FIRST SPOKE TO MARY NELSON in 1996, about ten minutes after I had received my first LaStone Therapy treatment. We talked for a while but she was just about to leave for the airport to teach a course. It took me until 1998 to get my act together, and through a set of coincidences, good fortune and circumstance, I did my LaStone training with her. This is her story.

Mary Dolores Nelson was born in Tucson, Arizona on 14 September, 1954. She was the middle child of five children, an older brother and sister and two younger brothers. She was raised in an Irish Catholic family that held true to the Irish Catholic traditions. Having met some of her siblings and heard stories about her parents, I believe this was clearly a wonderfully loving childhood, with huge amounts of love and fun.

They were the best parents anyone could ever ask for. Until their passing, old school-friends would stop by to see them and share what was going on in their lives. They imparted many gifts to many people throughout their time on this planet. I will miss them forever, even though I know they are with me whenever I call to them.

Christ and God were ever present in Mary's upbringing. Coming from Irish origins, there were many nuns and priests visiting with stories and gifts to enrich her beliefs.

I was most fortunate to meet nuns and priests that came from Ireland, bringing with them the gifts of exploring self and God through drawings and song. When I was a young teenager we would gather for weekend workshops designed to open our hearts to Jesus with drumming ceremonies, expression of the self with paper and pen, and long periods of silence, for internal journeys of our soul. Many of the traditional Catholic ceremonies were held outside, securing my beliefs in God and Mother Earth.

In my early years I would travel to the reservation with my mother, who did volunteer work with many of the Native American women. My first experience with death was at the age of seven when my very best friend took ill and began the process of passing into the next world. I would often see elders outside their small, grass-roof home singing and dancing. My mum told me not to bother them; that they were saying prayers for Rachael. As the days and weeks passed Rachael lost more and more weight, and her once-brown skin turned pale in colour. Our favourite last game we played was each day I would measure her wings by placing my small hand in her shoulder blades and then showing her how big her wings had grown overnight. Neither of us ever thought that she was losing so much weight due to the leukaemia that was the cause of her bones protruding as they did. We only knew her wings were growing so that when she did finally die she would be ready to fly. I never questioned this to be fact; you see, I had been talking to Blessed Mary for many years now. For me angels and saints were very real, and my best friend was becoming an angel right before my eyes.

As a young woman, Mary began to study metaphysical beliefs in addition to maintaining her Catholic faith. This combination sometimes caused problems and her family tried to 'help her' with her faith.

It wasn't long after Rachael's passing that the time came for me to be silent in regard to my on-going experiences with angels and spirits. My Aunt Betty had be hospitalised for talking to people who weren't there and I knew I would be next if I continued to speak about what I was seeing. So for the next twenty-eight years I chose not to speak about what I saw or heard from my guides. In those days I did not know for sure who they were. I gave them names associating them with Christian saints and angels. Then a time came in my late thirties when I saw them more as spirit guides than saints.

Mary's ability to combine her metaphysical experiences with her Catholic beliefs without compromising either also enabled her to study Native American cultures. This combination brought about her ability to remain spiritually, energetically and physically 'in touch' in her life, and was probably the key to her being able to receive the teachings of the stones from her spirit guide.

Now as I travel to the end of my forties I see my guides as an extension of the vibrating force of the universe; a universe that encompasses all life and all it has offered to humanity.

Mary left school wanting to become a vet but was unable to take the course. She therefore studied interior design and dress design in college. Some time after this, Mary found herself managing a health store in Tucson, Arizona. At the same time she undertook a course in massage at the now famous Desert Institute for Healing Arts (DIHA) in Arizona and graduated with honours. The training course she took opened up a whole new world of energy work, not just by the actual study but through her intuitive need to do more than just follow the 'stroke sheets'.

> I graduated from massage school in 1991. Throughout the fourteen months it took me to complete the 1,000-hour programme that DIHA offered, I heard about energy work and heard the word chakra and saw t'ai chi being done. However, my Catholic upbringing held me back, and the deep-seated fear of being a witch kept me from exploring any of these teachings. It was not until I was in my final term at massage school that I took a course in shiatsu for fourteen weeks. There I learned about chakras; I found the flow of energy going through me to be a joy and did not have to fear at least this part of myself.
>
> As soon as I began my homework and my own private practice away from school, and the Stroke Sheets we had to perform to pass each class, I began to play with energy work.
>
> I had no formal training except for the shiatsu programme at school. Yet my whole being knew deep within my soul that body-work was about blending the soul with the body. So I kept playing with that – how to approach the body, how to leave the body, how to move energy over the body. Somewhere inside me I knew that there was much more to this massage stuff than muscle and bone. I wanted to play with my clients, and play I did.

Throughout this period, Mary started to develop some of the techniques for her massage practice that have now become fundamental to the LaStone Therapy treatment we know today. Opening and Closing Spiral, Spinal Spiral, 'Up the left and Down the right' – these techniques have all become mantras to any therapist who has studied LaStone Therapy. The terminology may not be familiar, but the research Mary has subsequently done and the sharing of these experiences has shown us that they have origins that are nearly as old as the stones themselves.

Over a period of two and a half years I found ways in which to move around the table, 'up the left and out the right'. The comments I received as I continued to practise and explore the response of the body only confirmed my belief that we are spirited beings in a physical body that needs to be connected to its soul. Massage was the ticket to allow me to explore what the body and soul wanted of one another.

About six months or so before the stones came to me, I was practising ways in which to move up the body while holding the joints. I had heard about polarity and had not had the time or money to go to a workshop. So I was practising with my clients what felt best. I am very grateful to all my initial clients, who humoured me as I tried this or that on them. They let me know what felt good and what felt like nothing or triggered no response within their bodies.

I had been playing with energy on or over the body for about six months before the stones came to me. I experimented on my own with no guidance other than that of my clients and their responses to what I was doing. Through trial and error we found our way around the body and through the energy field, learning as we did so what each client liked or responded to in a positive way.

After qualifying, Mary went on to practise massage and very soon built a strong and successful practice. So much so, that as with many therapists she was beginning to feel the strain that comes with working on other people every day of the week. No matter how anatomically correct you try to be, damage will always occur to the muscles you use so regularly. Any therapist reading this book will know only too well the feeling of aching joints and potential damage to the fingers and thumbs that comes with repeated use, no matter how many precautions they take. As a therapist Mary found this difficult to overcome. The desire to do the best work for her clients combined with the pain felt after just a few treatments, with many more bookings to fulfil before the day was over.

It was in August 1993 that all this changed. On 19 August, 1993 Mary listened to her inner teacher speak to her about the stones and how to use them. At the time, she had an injury to her right shoulder that caused a lot of pain, and she needed a method that would be easier on her and beneficial to her clients.

LaStone Therapy came to me in the summer of 1993, while my niece Tonya Council-Bucinell and I were sitting in a sauna, staring at the hot rocks that were heating the entire room. I was struggling with a recurring shoulder injury and needed some type of extra help when working on trigger points in my clients. I silently asked Spirit [Mary's spirit guide] why I was in so much pain and how I could do massages with this shoulder.

The first message I received from Spirit was, 'Use the stones'. Use them for what? was my first thought. Then my mind went back to the pain in my shoulder. How was I going to massage Tonya, who was in my office for a treatment? I worried about causing myself more debilitating pain. Again the voice said, 'Use the stones.' I listened a little, but took no action. As we were leaving to do the massage, the voice called out louder, 'Pick up the stones and use them.' How could I ignore that voice? It was loud and clear what Spirit wanted. I chose two palm-sized stones and dropped them into a pot of ginger fomentation to use on Tonya. I found that mild pressure was enough to release her tense muscles. The heat and weight of the small stones did it all, saving me painful extra effort, and allowing my shoulder to rest and heal.

I longed to have the stones placed on my body, to feel their healing powers work their magic on me. I began to take time every day to lie with the stones. I did layouts on my body similar to the ones we do when we build castles of stones on each other during a workshop. With this type of energy work on myself, more messages began to come through even faster than when I am working with the stones in my hands on a client.

With each day's work, I was intuitively led to use more stones, and developed a method of progressively opening up the energy channels of the body, as well as working more deeply into the muscles with each application. As I began to grow with the stones I longed to know the voice that continued to speak to me from my inner teacher deep within my heart. I asked Spirit to guide me and knew without doubt that I would be shown how to find this Spirit that speaks to me. I prepared my body with the stones and I asked for this to be made clear to me. As soon as I placed the last stone on my third eye, I drifted off, out of body, not aware of time or space.

I began to see Joe (my husband) and myself on Salt River in Arizona, a place we both love to visit. Joe was fishing and I was doing what I always do when I am outside – collecting stones. It wasn't long before I got cold, so Joe made a fire and went back to camp to get my coat. I stayed back to continue collecting stones. Everywhere I go I collect stones. They call out to me. I saw beauty before me as I was harvesting my stones, with trees all around and grass to lie down upon. As I stepped into the river to gather a few more stones, I felt a presence nearby. Turning, I saw what appeared to be a Native American. I say this, because I grew up in Tucson, Arizona, and as a child was blessed with seeing many Native Americans dressed in their finest. This one was on a large brown horse and motioned to me, and asked, 'What are you doing?' No words were spoken. I just began to show with my hands the stones I was collecting. Then I walked over to the fire and cooked the stones in a make-believe bowl. Taking the stones off the fire, I rubbed my body with them and then handed him a stone. He put his hand out and took the stone, looking at me and the stone, then he again held out his hand and helped me up on to the horse with him.

Off we went down the river. There was so much beauty in front of us and the day seemed unending. He stopped near a large part of the river where the water was almost still. I got down and every stone I saw was the perfect stone for my work. I looked up at him and nodded, my eyes shining with delight like those of a child on Christmas morning. I marvelled at the beauty of stone after stone, and carefully placed each one on the river bank. Soon my pile of stones filled my heart and I knew I had enough for now. I looked around for the Spirit who had brought me to this place of abundance. There was no sign of him, but I knew in my heart he had been with me.

Then a thought came to me: 'Where was I and how was Joe going to find me?' Just then, Joe came up to me and handed me my coat. I was shocked. How did he know where I was? As I asked him, I realised that I was still in the place where he had left me. Everything was the same as before, except that my pile of perfect stones was there, waiting for me. I then realised that the Spirit that had taken me on that long ride down the beautiful river, had taken me through time, not space. I told Joe about my journey and gave thanks to Grandfather and Grandmother for the blessings of the day.

As I awoke from my self-treatment and remembered the joy and blessings that were set before my eyes and mind, I slowly removed the cooled stones from my body, giving thanks for each one and the messages they, and Spirit, had shared with me that day.

Later that night, as I was settling in for sleep, I again asked to have the voice of Spirit be known to me. When I awoke around 3.00 a.m., I went to my computer, as I do a lot, for I seem to listen to Spirit best in the early morning hours, when life is still in my house, the phone isn't ringing and the children aren't in need of my attention.

As I sat there with my fingers on the keys I began to type letters, and the voice said, 'No that's not it.' Again, letters found their way on to the screen, 'No that's not it,' again and again, until I heard, 'Yes, that is my name.' The name on the screen was San Juanette. I was not sure how to pronounce the name, so I repeated it over and over again until I heard, 'That's it' (San Juan ney). I was finally satisfied with the answer Spirit blessed me with on that early September morning.

San Juanette, Blessed Mary, Jesus, and all the angels and saints are a real part of who I am. They are as real to me as any physical being that has ever walked this planet. I call to them throughout the day and welcome the gifts they offer me. I am forever grateful for this internal knowledge of who I am in the unfolding universe.

With each day more messages came to Mary through her spirit guide. Her knowledge of the stones began to grow and develop into her very special treatment. Originally Mary called the treatment she was doing 'Hot Stone Massage', but very soon she was using cold stones as well. It was totally appropriate that she then decided to ask San Juanette what name to give this type of bodywork.

I first called this form of bodywork Hot Stone Massage (along with many variations of that). In a very short time I began to incorporate cold stones into my work. No longer was the name Hot Stone Massage enough to complement what I was accomplishing in my work with my clients. I again went to bed and asked for guidance from San Juanette. I asked 'What do you want to call what I am doing with the stones?' When 3.00 a.m. rolled around my sleep was again disturbed. As I got out of bed I heard 'LaStone Therapy'. I thought, 'How do I spell that one?' The answer came quickly. Now this form of bodywork had a name. I felt complete and satisfied with knowing that all was as it should be and that I was moving in the direction of Spirit. I give thanks to Great Grandfather and Great Grandmother for being by me at all times and speaking to me, so that I heard their most beloved words.

And so LaStone Therapy was born, but it didn't stop there. Mary began to incorporate the energy work she had experimented with in her early days as a student. Over a long period of refinement she developed the treatment as we know it now.

One day, I gave a stone treatment to a Healing Touch Instructor, Mary Hart. When the treatment was completed Mary asked me when I had studied Healing Touch and with whom. I said I never had and did not know what it was. She then asked when I had studied Brugh Joy's work and again I said that I knew nothing about it. Mary then explained to me that what I was trying to do with energy work is very similar to Healing Touch and Brugh Joy's work. She suggested that I start taking workshops in Healing Touch so that I could refine what I was working on and begin to understand what was happening within the body. Mary could tell I was guided to work in the field, yet she could also tell I knew nothing of what was truly happening to the client other than what the client was sharing with me, of feeling good and relaxed. So, with Mary Hart's willingness to trade with me the cost of a workshop, I went to my first Healing Touch workshop about a year later, and then attended workshops for two more levels. It was within these workshops that I saw the energy work I had been playing with fine tuned, and it was there that I found ways in which to understand what was happening, and why one treatment did this for a client and another one did something else.

I also bought *Joy's Way* by W. Brugh Joy, M.D., and studied his teachings. I was very pleased with the exercises at the back of his book. Barbara Brennan's books *Hands of Light* and *Light Emerging* were hard for me to fully understand. I am still to this day reading them over and over again.

Two years after my first workshop in Healing Touch and learning about Brugh Joy, a student at one of my workshops said to me, 'I know Brugh personally. Would you like his home address?' I said that of course I would, and went straight home and wrote Mr. Joy a letter introducing myself and explaining much of what I have just shared with you. I sent him a copy of the notes for LaStone instruction (I think I had about 100 pages back in 1995). Brugh wrote back and encouraged me to continue my studies, and gave me permission to use what I wanted out of his book. We spent many days writing backwards and forwards via e-mail, and I was very honoured that Mr. Joy took the time to write and assist me in understanding more of what

I had intuitively channelled twenty years after he had channelled it into his awareness.

You see Brugh was awakened to this work in 1973. I was awakened to its power in 1993. This is confirmation for me that when I hear messages from my guides they are bringing to my awareness a consciousness that expands the times of our planet. Over and over again I have found evidence that I channel in information that is aeons old, and years down the road I stumble across history that substantiates what I know in my heart to be true and righteous for the body, the mind and the soul. I am forever grateful and honoured to be willing to hear the messages my guides have to offer me. I am forever willing to share these teachings with others.

Very soon, with this potent combination of stone work and energy work, Mary's clients were filling her booking lists until she could no longer satisfy the demand for this amazing treatment. Mary was incredibly busy but was also able to carry on her treatments, balancing and healing her clients with no physical damage to herself. Pretty soon it was clear that she would have to find a way to make LaStone Therapy more widely available to both clients and other therapists – clients so that they could benefit from the effects of the therapy, and therapists so that they could protect themselves and extend their working lives and livelihoods.

Over time Mary trained her good friends and fellow therapists. Tomi Wertheim was one of the first people Mary enrolled to promote the teachings of the stones and the LaStone treatment. She shared the therapy with Patricia Warren, her hydrotherapy instructor at the Desert Institute. Patricia's expertise enabled Mary to understand initially and then study further the effects of the different temperatures she was using – the thermotherapy. Patti Templin, on the other hand, worked with Mary and the stones to develop the energetic and healing aspects of the treatment. Next came Teri Williams, a Reiki Master and rebirthing therapist. Over the next few years Mary developed the knowledge required to understand the full potential of this treatment by introducing to it therapists qualified in hugely diverse areas.

Not only has the knowledge developed but so has the geography. LaStone instructors are now to be found worldwide. From humble beginnings in 1993 there are now over twenty-two Original Body LaStone instructors and several more speciality instructors teaching courses such as Beyond Basics, Deep Tissue, Stone Chi Therapy, Stone Facials, Stone Soul Connection, Dances with Stones, Simply Stones, Simply Beauty and Not Just Polished Stones. All of these are explained later in the book in greater detail.

## CHAPTER THREE

# How I Came to LaStone

M Y STORY IS A SIMILAR SET of coincidences, amazing expe-riences and things that just should not have happened to any one person. That is, unless you believe that there is another force or energy which is in charge of what we get up to, rather than that we are the pilots to our destinations.

Every time I teach a course, I am faced by a room full of people, each of whom has their own story to tell about how they came to be there. Some are obviously sent by their spas, and the amount of hugely successful spas that make LaStone an integral part of their in-house training is a testament to the treatment itself. Others have been waiting to find a suitable date, and others still have been reading about the treatment and have eventually decided to make the investment. But nearly every student has a story that shows how stones or nature have been a very important part of their life, long before they had heard about LaStone Therapy. It is almost as if the treatment was waiting to happen in their lives. They were just a second away from it in everything they did, but the time had to be right, as well as the course itself.

Well, just as my experiences happened with LaStone, my experiences with everything else since then have opened me up to realising that things happen for a reason. Like it or not, things happen and we end up doing things we wouldn't dream of doing and things we wouldn't have thought were possible.

In 1996 I was working as a massage therapist and looking to add some power to my treatment, to take it to another level. The limitations of my hands were not enough. I had introduced the use of linen mitts to cool my clients' 'pumped-up' muscles after I had been working them. I was dabbling in oils to get deeper into the relaxation, but I was feeling really frustrated that I couldn't do more.

I wasn't yet at the stage where my muscles were getting damaged, but more frustrated and bored by what I was doing. I needed to get deeper, quicker and more effectively.

At this time I received a call from a friend whom I hadn't heard from for a while and this slightly worried me, as the last conversation we had had, the last time we had met, implied that things were not all well with her. This turned out to be the case. Without going into details, my good friend had found herself in the most dreadful situation in her life. It was awful – one of those situations where you want to help, but no matter what you say or do it does not ease the pain that you know the person must be going through. Not only that, but you cannot see how anyone could ever come back from such a situation.

My friend's boss seemed to be going through the very same thought process that I was and she decided that the best place to be was a spa in Tucson, Arizona, which she had recently visited. Not only was this a chance to step away and to try to gain some form of perspective on the situation, but she also clearly knew that it would be one of those life-changing experiences that was required at the time. Not wishing her to travel alone, she said she would fund a trip for two people for ten days.

At that time I had recently set up a school and clinic for massage therapy with a friend and was busy, but not every day. I had previously worked in a job where I would never have been able to take an extended break without several months' notice. My recent and very unexpected career change had made me much more flexible.

I got a phone call asking me if I could travel at short notice. Well, how much encouragement does a girl need? I was fine to take the time, happy to be with my friend and looking forward to an experience of a lifetime. Due to circumstances, we were both able to do this without much notice, time or even thought.

There were a few conditions to our visit. We were told that once we were there we had to make sure we attended something called 'Quantum Leap'. We needed to book into 'Equine Experience' and we were also to make sure we had a LaStone Therapy treatment – something to do with massage with hot and cold stones. Well, there didn't seem to be too much problem with any of these requirements, so off we went.

During the trip we had amazing experiences. Every day we did something that was totally unreal, something that would never normally have entered our lives. My friend's boss was exactly right; this was the place to be to reassess your life, to explore your potential and to make decisions about how to move forward. It was also far enough away to get some real perspective on things.

It also became apparent that the challenges we had been set were just that. Quantum Leap turned out to be jumping off a twenty-five-foot-high telegraph pole with nothing but trust and a few harnesses to keep you alive. Just climbing the pole step by step had us both virtually in tears of fear and excitement, but with the gentle cooperation of the team we made it to the top. Once there, there was the small issue of letting go of the stranglehold you had on each of the steps and standing upright on what felt like a very small side plate – which wobbled! I think you get the picture.

The next day we did Equine Experience, which was just unbelievable. Not only did we walk safely UNDER a horse's stomach and hug its bottom (yes, everything we are taught never to do for safety's sake), but we also groomed a horse, learnt respect for it and then, using breathing, body language and the power of thought, we got the horse to trot, canter and gallop. We were horse whispering. If you ever get the chance to be in a ring with just you and a horse, all the time in the world and the most understanding instructor you can ever conceive, then the experience of being one with the mind of one of these amazing creatures will truly change your life. The emotion of connection with yourself is unimaginable. Taking this training into your own life from the ring is hugely humbling and at the same time totally empowering.

So, when the only challenge left was to have LaStone Therapy, we were getting pretty sure that there was nothing that could have an effect on us any more – we were already empowered beyond belief.

What can I say? As a massage therapist I was trying to have a treatment. Booking in for treatments when you do them for a living is an odd experience. You want the treatment because you really need it but you want to stay alert and aware so that you can see or feel what the therapist is doing. Well, this treatment was impossible to stay with. All I knew was that once the treatment was completed I had no option but to learn how to become a LaStone therapist. In my mind I had seen that there was no other way to work. The stones were so penetrating and therapeutic, my mind was so enlivened but calm, and my spirit was soaring – so I thought, get me to a class right now!

I asked the therapist how they had learned to do this therapy. The reply was one of those things you don't ever expect to hear. 'Mary Nelson originated this treatment and she lives just down the road in Tucson; here is her telephone number – give her a call.'

I went to my room and gave Mary a call. She was in the process of packing for a trip to California to teach, but we discussed the possibility of her coming to the UK to teach at the school we had opened. We talked some more and left it at that.

After the trip my friend and I returned renewed and refreshed. It had been an experience that we still hold good in our hearts today. I left thinking I would love to return some day and that it would be great to pay back my friend for the experience she had shared with me. I have no doubt that it helped her to make the steps back into her life with a little more certainty and a measure of confidence that you wouldn't have dreamt was possible had you been through what she had. The experience she allowed me to share with her changed us both.

I was so empowered and fired up that I decided I was going to write a book. This sounds glib, but for months I had been handing out bits of A4 paper to my clients, with instructions about how to eat healthily and cleanse, but now I decided it was time to put all this together into a book. I wrote to various publishers with my idea and got back into the swing of daily life. I thought about LaStone often but didn't get around to picking up the phone to make the booking.

The book project did take off. After a few unsuccessful meetings with publishers, I eventually signed a contract with my current publisher, Piatkus Books. I had always thought that if I did get to write a book and if it did actually earn me any money, I would use that money to take myself, my friend and some other friends back to Tucson. This was a secret to be shared. In my mind, if everyone could have the same experience that we had had, then everyone's lives would be enriched. Put that together with the fact that it would be an amazing experience to go through the same thing with a group of girl friends and it would be a total blast.

Two years later, my first royalty cheque came through. Together with my friend and two others we made the return trip to Tucson. I thought about doing the LaStone training but it simply passed through my mind, as many thoughts do when you are busy. Then I got a call from one of my fellow travellers asking whether I had seen this month's *Tatler* magazine. I found a copy, and there in the middle was a picture of the basalt stones and a very short article describing LaStone Therapy, how it was the hottest treatment in American spas and how, as the journalist put it, 'we eagerly await its arrival on these shores'.

If that wasn't a kick up the backside then I don't know what was. This journalist was stating in black and white that it was huge in the States and now we wanted it to be huge over here. Right there and then, I decided that I wanted to be a LaStone therapist. I wanted to introduce a new and amazingly therapeutic treatment into my clinic and into the UK, and I wanted to eventually become an instructor. Our expanding school could offer something quite different from all the other schools around. I saw my opportunity to do something really different. My friend pointing out the article had given me the push to sort things out.

I added some days to my trip and did my training in Jacksonville, Florida in September 1998.

I launched the treatment in October 1998 and my clinic was extremely busy from day one. A year later Mary came to the UK, and I did my instructor's training with her. I started the training courses in the UK expecting them to grow slowly, but they were very busy from day one. I remember saying to Mary that I would like to teach small groups at the start and she laughed. She clearly knew how busy I was about to be and how much in demand this treatment was going to be. And this has been the case.

While I was getting involved in LaStone I continued to write. At the same time I was contacted by a man in Chile. He had recently had a LaStone treatment in Mexico and had seen my name on the website. He wanted copies of my books to be sent to him. I am now involved in setting up a destination spa in Chile and opening some amazing day spas in Chile and other parts of South America.

My main subject for writing has been Detox, but my publisher heard about LaStone and that is why I am now able to write this book.

LaStone Therapy enables people to change their lives. The connections are brilliant:

- I had a friend.
- I had a clinic.
- I had the time.
- I went away on a trip to Tucson.
- I had a LaStone treatment.
- I had never been to America.
- I felt empowered to write a book.
- My book was successful enough to raise the cash to go back to Tucson.
- A magazine article happened to appear just before this second trip.
- I booked my training.
- I launched the treatment in the UK.
- I got my instructor's certificate.
- I taught the course at my school.
- I put the course on the website.
- A man in Chile saw the website.
- The man had had a treatment and read my books.
- I am now a shareholder in a spa group in South America.
- I am writing this book because my publisher for Detox was happy to publish a book on LaStone.
- I am training in a new therapy next year because the instructor of the course was on one of my courses.

The opportunities just never cease to amaze me.

I say to my students that this treatment can give you anything you want it to, that it opens up your horizons and that things you never thought possible become normal.

## CHAPTER FOUR

# How LaStone Therapy Works

A TRUE LASTONE THERAPY TREATMENT involves many, many aspects. We will go on to learn about each aspect of the treatment in detail, but here is a description of what may take place in a full hour-and-a-quarter LaStone Therapy treatment.

## What Happens During a Treatment

You lie on a massage couch with either no clothes on or wearing simply your briefs. You are covered with a towel and made to feel warm and comfortable. The therapist collects a selection of heated and cooled stones and brings them to the head of the table. You sit up and the therapist carefully places the stones on the table, where either side of your spine will be, so that they will work on every section of your back muscles. The stones are covered and you are rolled down onto them. Any adjustments are made and then a pillow stone is placed under your neck and tucked under the base of your skull – just where you hold all the tension.

The therapist is then likely to place stones in the palms of your hands, wrapped so that they are not too hot at first. The treatment has begun. Stones are removed from the hot tank or cooler and then placed on the table, next to your leg. The therapist carries out some energy work that is called the Opening Spiral. This is to relax you and open you energetically so that the therapist can work within your auric field. This means that you will feel the effects of a much deeper and more profound treatment.

Then the stones are placed along the front of your body on your key chakra points, or energy points. This is done while the therapist is doing energy connection work for proper stone placement. Each limb is connected as each stone is placed. The chakras also correlate with comfortable places along the front of your body.

Once the stones are placed the therapist starts a process of massaging hot and cool stones on your body, legs, toes, arms, neck, shoulders and face. The massage can be firm or light, but it is delivered through the beautiful stones. Toe stones can be slipped between each toe, and hot stones can be worked over each and every facial muscle. Knots and tension disappear from your neck, and your shoulders and hands are worked to relax and stretch them.

Once the work is complete on the front of your body, it is time to work on the back. The therapist slowly removes the stones from the top of your body, using each of your breaths as an indicator of when to pick up a stone. Once all the stones have been removed the therapist completes the energy work for this side of the body and commences the closing spiral. This puts you back together, grounds you and makes you feel safe.

You are asked to sit up slowly and once the stones have been removed from under you, you may roll over to find an amazing stone in a fabric cover to lie your tummy on. You are covered by the towel now but lying on your front. Your ankles are supported by a pillow. The therapist carries out energy connection again on each leg and arm, and along the spine. While doing the connection, a stone is placed on your sacrum or lower back, and stones in a soft fabric tube are draped around your neck.

Again, the massage takes place and each and every muscle can be worked. The back has been lying on those stones for the first half of the treatment, so the muscles will melt under the careful and skilful work of the therapist. Certain strokes are deeper, under the scapula and resonating deep through your rib cage, but the end result will leave you feeling amazing.

Once the massage is complete the towel is used to cover you again and the therapist uses a piece of Chinese flourite crystal to do the Spinal Spiral strokes to ground and centre you once more.

After the Spinal Spiral, your hands and feet are washed and essential oils are applied to them. A number of things may then happen, but most often a selection of beautiful Tibetan bowls will be placed along your spine and chimed so that the resonance travels deep into your body, demonstrating that your muscles are totally relaxed as you feel the sound waves travel unhindered around your body. Then Native American wild sage is used to smudge or clear the energy around your body and in the room. This is called neutralising, and we use an abalone shell and a fabulous fan of feathers for it. The sage is lit and the therapist travels around your body to complete the treatment.

The sheet you are lying on is then wrapped around you for comfort and security while you return to this world and the room you are in.

Your therapist will either leave you or bring you some water or a tisane to refresh you and prepare you for the world outside.

## How the Treatment Feels – Some Testimonials

So, after all that, what do people get from LaStone Therapy? What are they saying? One of the overriding responses to a LaStone Therapy treatment is that it is much, much more than a simple treatment. Each client finds something different, and each treatment for the same person is totally different. Some people will feel the heat, others talk of the deep relaxation, and many talk of nurturing, grounding and centring. Clients report sensations of invigoration and increased energy. Many see colours or visions, and some have relatives that have passed away visit them in their relaxed state. Some feel their bodies spinning, and some simply find it the deepest, most thorough massage they have ever experienced. There is no 'take it or leave it' aspect to LaStone. Here are some reports from both therapists and clients, starting with a summary from Mary Nelson.

In the following few paragraphs, I've tried to condense the feedback I've been getting from my clients during the various stages of my massage using stones. 'Sinking into the Earth' and 'feeling cradled by Mother Earth' have been surprisingly common responses. The client seems to be in some sort of reverie or deep meditative state by the end of the massage, more often than with regular massage techniques.

'Trails of heat are flowing deep within my body, flowing upwards from my feet, through my legs, and swirling all over my back, lingering just long enough to melt the tension from each muscle. As the stones give up their heat, I find them resting in the palms of my hands, and I sink into the table, grounded in Mother Earth. More hot stones now travel up the same paths as before, staying a little longer, their heat penetrating a little deeper, working out a few stubborn trigger points. Again, these stones find their way to my palms, replacing those that have now cooled.

'Once again, fresh stones, radiant with heat, chase the last bits of tension from my muscles, like beaming Sun rays melting their way through chunks of ice. I have been bathed in heat.

'Turning over is an effort. Now I feel these hot stones resting on my front chakras, opening and softening each one. Another caresses the back of my neck. These stones have become a part of me. As the massage continues, I dissolve into dreamtime, a world of fantastic colours and visions, allowing Mother Earth to heal me in body, mind and spirit, knowing I am one with all things, and that this is good.

'As the cooling stones are lifted from each chakra, I feel a lifting of my spirit as well. I let go of the burdens I have been carrying. I feel light, buoyant, balanced, centred and cradled. I am whole again.'

To truly learn the art of LaStone Therapy, one must receive the treatment from a skilled practitioner and take the workshops taught by Mary Nelson or one of her certified instructors. The simple act of transferring one stone to another from hand to foot must be done with rhythm and grace, giving the client a feeling of dancing with the stones, a joining of their body with the stones in a rhythmical movement, and a reconnection with their roots to Mother Earth. This text is designed as an aid to therapists who practise LaStone Therapy. In order to become skilled at this powerful treatment one must go beyond this book, to the way LaStone Therapy feels on your own body. Watch as Mary performs this most powerful treatment at one of her workshops. All these tools together may enable you to become a LaStone therapist with great skill, and intuitiveness.

*Margaret Avery-Moon, Therapist, Director and Owner of Desert Institute of the Healing Arts, Massage Therapy School, Tucson, Arizona, USA.*

I walked into the treatment with a headache and my shoulders tucked under my earlobes. I was a woman in search of immediate relief, and that's pretty much what I got.

*Julia Carling, Journalist, Client, UK.*

Unlike a normal massage, the sense of warmth seemed to cover me rather than stay only in the place on my body where the therapist was currently working. The deep push of the long, slow strokes was pleasantly disorientating.

As I felt the stones touching my body, images from my childhood flashed through my mind, from the smell of the honeysuckle creeping through my open window at home on a summer evening to the cobalt flash of a kingfisher flying by as I skimmed stones across the river. I emerged into a spring afternoon feeling refreshed, as if the world around me was balmy. I may not have had visions or communicated with any spirit guides, but my body felt more fluid and more connected with the Earth – somewhat as I imagine keen gardeners feel – rather than caught up in the whirl of day-to-day existence on its surface.

*Chris Taylor, Journalist, Client, UK.*

The LaStone massage is wonderfully warm, nurturing and very effective in melting away knots and stress in the body! Our guests love this new alternative to a regular massage!

*Scottsdale Princess, Therapist, Scottsdale, Arizona, USA.*

I just wanted something relaxing so I took myself off for a LaStone treatment. I thought it was wonderful. The massage with stones was like having warm wax poured all over your body. I had started to suffer from a frozen shoulder, and thought the heat of LaStone would be really soothing. A frozen shoulder can be related to carrying too many burdens mentally, as well as having physical causes, and can take up to a year to heal on its own. At the time I was doing shiatsu and a lot of political work about complementary therapies as well.

LaStone moved the stagnation in the sixth joint and was very restorative. The heat relieved the tension and the cool soothed the inflammation. As well as the physical work, I found the cold stone on the third eye – between my eyebrows – really cleared my mind too. I had three or four treatments on my shoulder, including two in one week, and my symptoms have cleared completely. I do believe illnesses are trying to teach you something. I've been simplifying my life recently, but the problem may have also taught me to be less cynical. I thought LaStone was just a strange new American fad, but now I'm a real fan.

*Katharine Hall, Client, UK.*

I am writing on behalf of The Boulders resort to report the smashing success of the 'Boulders Hot Rock Massage' (more commonly known as 'LaStone Therapy'). Our therapists and guests have thoroughly enjoyed this wonderful type of therapeutic work since The Boulders added it to our menu in '96.

Our guests have usually heard about the 'Hot Rocks' before they even arrive at The Boulders. Currently, your treatment is the most requested treatment at our resort. What a compliment to your innovative discovery!

Thank you for all the time and effort you have invested in The Boulders spa. We always boast the fact that we were one of the first spas in the country to offer this amazing therapy.

*The Boulders, Therapists, Carefree, Arizona, USA.*

We have spent the past eight years developing a very loyal following here in Lexington, Kentucky. This past year we started looking for some new services to offer to our valuable clients, something new and different for them to enjoy.

We located Mary Nelson and were thrilled with the training provided to our therapists in LaStone Therapy. This has provided us with a fabulous new technique for our clients. We feel our continued growth and success this year has been complimented by this wonderful new therapy treatment. Our clients and our therapists love the LaStone treatments!

*Lexington's Profession Massage Center Inc., Therapists, Lexington, Kentucky, USA.*

During LaStone Therapy I feel 'at home'. The vibration of the stones interacts with my energy field in such a manner as to facilitate the release of energies which I no longer wish to hold. On a physical level, the warmth or coolness of the stones feels wonderful; the stones are healing tools which are great adjuncts to massage and energy work. The heaviness of the stones adds a feeling of physical security, as well as emotional security. The stones facilitate healing at all levels, from basic physical healing to emotional, mental and spiritual healing.

*Valerie Sorrells, Client, USA.*

A client had called complaining of lower back pain, which happened that morning. As I was looking at my stones I thought 'Why not ice them?' A half-hour before the appointment time, I poured four cups of ice over and around the stones. When the client came in, I was glad I had iced the stones. He could hardly move, much less get up on my table. Due to possible spinal problems (his chiropractor was closed for the weekend), I couldn't apply much pressure. The weight of the stones was minimal and while I was constantly turning them and doing an effleurage stroke the client had no discomfort. When I felt the cold leaving the stones I exchanged them for another set. The client had no discomfort from the deepening cold and the results were great. He had walked in all bent over, and he walked out standing straight up. Two days later he came in again, much better, but still sore. I started with heated stones and ended with iced. After four treatments in a week he jumped into my massage room and thanked me profusely. It was the quickest he had ever healed.

I also work for a chiropractor and have used LaStone Therapy on clients who have been in car accidents and whose muscles have contracted from extensive pain. With the gentle pressure of the stones the muscles relax and the spine can be adjusted more easily.

*Kathy Kay, Therapist, USA.*

As soon as I lay down on the stones, I went into a state of deep relaxation – the heat penetrating my body felt amazing. It reminded me of walking on warm sands on the beach with the Sun shining on my back. The stones positioned on my body were of different sizes and some, especially the one on my stomach, felt heavy, but it was a nice, comforting weight – like a hot-water bottle.

I thought the stones would feel incredibly rough on my skin, but they were incredibly smooth – like flesh on flesh. Rachel massaged my entire body with a stone in each hand and really focused on my problem areas – I could literally feel the knots unravelling. After the treatment I felt suprisingly energised – like I could go out and get on with the rest of the day.

*Sarah Quarton, Client, London, UK.*

The stones are a wonderful part of massage, allowing relaxation to take over quickly. I will only utilise a therapist who has this training in their resume.

The use of the stones with massage therapy allows the receiver to relax more fully. It really works wonderfully! All I can think to say is the stones are fantastic. I can say I will only have the stone therapy as my massage of choice.

*Mona Wright, Client, USA.*

The stones feel like 'Friends'. They give an immediate comfort of warmth and relaxation, the minute they touch my skin. I also like the smooth texture of the stones, especially when wet. The velvet texture of the wet stones mixing with the oil sliding over my skin is a unique feeling.

It's luxurious and powerful, causing great relief of tension and pressures. Mary's combination of styles and stones works for me! I highly recommend 'LaStone Therapy'.

*Gigi Brown, Client, USA.*

I can't imagine massage without the warmth and healing power of the stones. You don't feel uncomfortable lumps on your back when lying on them; you don't feel the weight from them resting on top of you either. You just feel absolutely balanced, comforted, cradled in all the right places. They seem to absorb all the aches and pains and you become one with the stones; you just don't know they are there. I have to examine them afterwards just so I know what size stone was placed and where it was. My body craves the warmth I get from the stones, which is as important as is the massage. Some of my favourite placements of the stones are: the ones that go between my toes, the one that cradles my neck, and the ones that I hold in my hands. The stones have healing powers as well as their comforting warmth. They are magical!

*Donna Wasley, Client, UK.*

LaStone Therapy takes massage to different levels in my bodywork. Not only does the heat from the stones provide a warm, nurturing massage, but the stones enable the massage therapist to work at deeper levels than may be possible with just the hands. I have experienced the movement of deeper healing energies and a release of emotional issues that I had been holding onto for a long time. At first I couldn't imagine how lying on stones could possibly be comfortable, then I experienced their power and nurturing gentleness! I would highly recommend LaStone Therapy to everyone.

*Valerie Barsevich, Client, USA.*

I would like to inform anyone reading this letter of the effectiveness and the beauty of the massage I was given by Mary Nelson. The professional manner and approach that were given to me were exemplary. The uniqueness of Mary's treatment with the inclusion of LaStone Therapy appears to be a very effective tool in the healing process. My compliments to her on the utilisation of nature's tools to heal people.

*Dr. Arnold A. Orbach, Chiropractic Physician, Client, USA.*

As a professional escape artist (one of only six full time in the world) and stunt man, my body is my equipment. I have several doctors who have advised me to use some form of massage therapy on a regular basis. Massage therapies are for healing the damage that my body receives and also act as a preventative measure ... helping me to keep my body in the best physical condition possible.

I have to be ready at a moment's notice to perform an escape, beneath a hot-air balloon or helicopter, without safety lines (authorized up to 30,000 feet). If I'm not ... I could die.

One of the best treatments for healing my body and keeping it from further injury has been LaStone Therapy treatment, administered to me by one of the nation's top massage therapists Sheena Paulus. I had tried a similar stone treatment previously, but it wasn't of the calibre of LaStone Therapy. It was also my first experience with cold stones and I was pleased with the results. Depending on the injury, it was great ... switching from cold to hot on different muscles made my pain disappear and improved my healing time tremendously.

I would recommend LaStone Therapy treatment to anyone seeking relief from pain or to prevent sports-related injuries. I am convinced LaStone Therapy is the Last One Therapy.

*Rick Maisel, Escape Artist, Client, USA.*

LaStone adds a fourth dimension, providing dynamically deep treatments for our clients. In the business of selling exceptionally good treatments, combining therapeutic and stress-relieving benefits, LaStone achieves more in a single treatment than most other 'hands-on' therapies.

LaStone gives our therapists greater results, combining the power of the stones, thermotherapy and deep massage. The therapeutic value is unparalleled.

LaStone achieves more benefit to a client in an hour and a half than many other treatments. It provides both therapeutic and customer satisfaction value. LaStone is more than a treatment.

*Fay Wancke, Therapist, Spa NK, London, UK.*

And then, if that was not enough to convince you, you may enjoy this extract from a well-known and very funny book about a woman who tried to find total enlightenment through therapeutic treatments. The treatment was carried out by myself when I first started working with LaStone Therapy and I did not know that the client was writing a book at the time. It seems she approved, anyway! The extract is from Isabel Losada's *The Battersea Park Road to Enlightenment*, published by Bloomsbury.

There is a way to be stoned that does not involve either the ancient punishment for adultery or the excess use of drugs or alcohol.

Yes, there is a form of massage known as LaStone.

I happened to see an article about this in the middle of my search for the ultimate massage and, although strictly speaking it wasn't part of the plan, I couldn't resist it. I have always been very partial to stones.

My home is full of them. You know those eccentric characters that are incapable of spending the day on the beach without robbing the natural environment of its riches and hobbling up the beach at the end of the day, pockets laden with rocks? Your narrator is one of them, it takes all sorts.

Now, you may wonder why anyone would want to be massaged with a rock when the human hand is surely softer. To discover the answer to this question I had to go to Harley Street, of all places. You wouldn't have thought that a street so prestigious for expertise in the medical field would have people getting silently stoned behind closed doors would you? But sure enough, there is a woman hiding there who does weird oily things with hot rocks.

I cycled from Battersea to Harley Street and arrived just in time for her to be ready with a glass of mineral water.

She looked rather medical, like a young nurse. I was getting used to taking my clothes off and lying on her pleasantly wide table I began to feel very happy.

She had filled the room with a wonderful Aromatherapy oil scent called energy. It made breathing a sensuous experience. And somewhere there was a tape playing plinky plonky New Age music.

The first part of this new experience involved sitting up and then lying down again onto a row of hot stones that had been laid out to heat up the muscles on either side of the spine. Damned clever. Don't you find that when you lie down on a stone beach, no matter how much you wriggle there is always a stone that insists on digging itself into your back? This was a blissful re-enactment of that experience. As I lay down on the stones each one was perfectly placed to match all the major muscle groups. I sighed, Oh yes, heat just there, and there and there. Then she put a round flat, hot stone wrapped in a sheet on to my stomach, and one on my breastbone. And one anywhere else where it wouldn't fall off. It was a great way to warm up.

One stone was put in the middle of my forehead and eight little stones were put between my toes. Then she took two large hot stones and gave them to me to hold. You may be thinking, this is all very well for people with nothing better to do with their time, but how do you know that there could be anything better?

You see, these crazy Americans have come up with a thousand and one ways to produce a feeling of bliss. Maybe it's something primal about stones but they do have something very reassuring about them. Holding a beautiful round stone in your hand does produce a feeling of being 'in touch' with reality somehow, doesn't it.

So, if you take that feeling and multiply it by the number of stones I was currently 'in touch' with, you can begin to imagine the effect of all this. Granted, I did feel a little daft. The days when I was dubious of the latest American fad to hit London were long gone. Now I just wanted to try them all, even if it did look as if someone was trying to bury me.

Then an oily stone started to massage my arm. I suppose her hand must have been connected to it at some point but I couldn't be sure. She was so skilful that it was hard to tell what was a stone and what was her hand, except that the stone was hotter. I began to feel a rush of affection for the stone. It was so good at massage. I'd had grown men in my life who claimed to be experienced lovers who couldn't make my arm feel as good as this stone could. Yes, I was fond of this rock.

She moved to work on the other arm. A new stone appeared in my life. As warm and tender as the last. It understood my new arm. It knew how to hollow itself round every tightened sinew. It knew how to slide itself along every aching tendon. My affection was growing deeper. I was interested in dating the stone.

There seemed to be battalions of them lined up to please me. No sooner had one cooled down than it was replaced by another. You are allowing them to give you their heat, she said.

Doesn't everyone? Surely I wasn't doing anything special. Some people do not receive the heat. They are resistant to it. With some clients I don't need to change the stones at all. Everyone is different.

Finally I have found something in life for which I have a talent. Receiving heat from the stones. Then some little pebbles started to make love to my face. They slid around happily. So intimate, so gentle. I wanted to proclaim my tenderness to them, Oh stones – how I do love thee.

Then I had to turn over. As I lay down there was a round flat stone that fitted perfectly into the pelvic girdle. It was like lying on a hot water bottle only twice as good and even quite sexy.

Heat was against the pubic bone. My potential new relationship was feeling very promising. And the uncanny feeling of being understood was becoming increasingly worrying. Maybe this is what I'd been doing wrong all these years. Trying to have relationships with people.

A stone started to express its devotion to my neck. I had a knotted muscle on the right-hand side that had been there for years. Many a masseur had skimmed straight over it. But not this stone. The heat was wonderful and the scented oil meant the stone could slide into the problem without being at all painful. I was lost. Oh yes, stone, yes. Where have you been all my life?

Then down my shoulders, and down my back. The stones pushed their way down onto my shoulder muscles as if trying to bury themselves. I said 'Ow', but I wasn't complaining. For my back, two twin stones slid up and down either side of my spine. They moved down my legs and started on my feet. So few men understand what an utter source of bliss the feet can be. Did you know that the tips of the toes like the tips of the fingers are amongst the most sensitive places in the body? The huge number of nerve endings in the fingertips is what makes it possible for the blind to learn Braille. We have hugely sensitive fingers. And toes. You may not know this but the rocks did.

A pebble was stroking my foot. There may once have been a man who had felt so passionate about the outside edge of my foot

... but I couldn't remember him. I was in love with this rock. So warm, so undemanding, so giving, so well rounded. Then the stones started to speak to me. Why are you always fighting your life and treating it as a struggle? Why are you always resistant? Why do you try so hard? Let things happen. Relax, be gentle. I was now being counselled by the stones. I was ready to make a commitment. It was going to have to be marriage. I take thee stone, to have and to hold from this day forth.

Then a terrible thing happened. A human voice spoke, 'Your session is now over.' Who was this silly woman, lie still for a while and then sit up slowly. She left the room. I lay feeling the flat, round stone warm against my tummy. I sat up and unwrapped it from its sheet. It was just a normal beach stone made of basalt but I loved it.

I wanted to take it home. But they are very spiritual things, rocks. Like nuns, they don't save their love for just one person but have a similar level of devotion to everyone they meet. Alas they would be just as attentive to the needs of the next customer. Blast non-attachment. I sighed and placed the rock lovingly on the massage bed.

As I put my clothes back on I felt like Celia Johnson in *Brief Encounter*. I had to leave, to return to my washing up. I walked courageously from the room. A new heroine for the new millennium. Isabel leaves rocks. Never let it be said that my life is not full of brave and heroic actions.

As I cycled home I remembered other meetings with rocks. The memory at my rebirthing of running over them to hurt my feet. Now I had made peace with them and they were yet one more lump in the universe which I held deep in affection. Gosh, accidental progress along the road to Enlightenment while in selfish pursuit of the ultimate massage. Sometimes, life is good.

Having read some of the feedback from clients and therapists alike, you can see that LaStone Therapy is truly different, hugely enjoyable and totally therapeutic.

## CHAPTER FIVE

# Stones Throughout the Ages

MANY PEOPLE SAY that LaStone Therapy is a Native American treatment. This is not strictly true. Native Americans did not, as far as we are aware, use stones in a massage practice. However, the roots of this therapy are so inextricably linked with the culture and beliefs of the Native Americans that the connection is easily explained. Their honour towards the Stone Clan People and the knowledge and teachings of stones is inextricable with their culture.

They respect all natural things – animals are called four-leggeds as we are called two-leggeds. Nature has an unquestionable value and respect for them. They would never for a moment think that we were anything other than subjects of nature rather than rulers.

The spirit guide that channelled the treatment to Mary Nelson was San Juanette, a Native American guide. Many of the techniques used in the treatment have their roots in Native American culture; the use of sage in cleansing and the invoking of spirits during the treatment are truly part of the culture.

What we are not saying (and we hope that no one misunderstands us) is that the Native American cultures practised LaStone Therapy. What we can see when we look at the history of healing stones is that the Native Americans embrace many of the values embodied in the LaStone treatment.

We are the students of this therapy; they are our masters.

# Stone Use Through the Ages

As mentioned before, there is nothing new about LaStone Therapy. It is a modern treatment embedded in ancient principles. What is new is the unique combination of many, many tried and tested elements.

Now that we have looked at how the treatment came about we can start to separate these individual elements and see what part they have to play in the whole.

## Stone cultures

The stones used in LaStone are probably the oldest part of the treatment – how does 4,600 million years old sound? The Earth is thought to be that old and so the rocks that are formed from its core are fairly close relatives. We use naturally shaped basalt pebbles and marble pebbles that have been cut to shape to deliver the hot and cold temperatures.

Before we look at the types of stone and why we use them, we can look at how other cultures have used stone to represent some of the most important aspects of their lives. Stone has been used for worship, knowledge and survival for millions of years.

In Native American tradition the Stone Clan People (stones) were the first beings to inhabit the Earth. They believed that stones, rocks and boulders hold the memory of every event that has occurred not only on this planet but also throughout the universe. They did not discern living creatures as non-human or inferior or even non-animal – indeed, the categories were simply two-leggeds, four-leggeds and plants. It is our cultures that have decided on our own superiority – that humans are better than animals and that we can own them.

In reality, we only need a short burst of heavy rain or the 'wrong kind of leaves on the line', or a little bit too much wind, to realise very swiftly that we are most definitely not in charge. When Mother Nature decides to remind us she is there we are left in no doubt about who has the upper hand.

## Introducing the Stone People

Stones have souls and spirits. If you start to understand this then you can start to see what may be the fifth element, the quintessence of LaStone Therapy. Respect for nature is all it really needs.

The following verse and words are written by Jamie Sams, a prolific author on Native American cultures and spirituality. The extract is from *Sacred Path Cards, The Discovery of Self Through Native Teachings*, published by HarperCollins.

> Stone People
> Record Holders of the Earth
> Will you please explain
> The history that gave us birth
> The truth you do contain?
>
> Like your cousins of the seas
> The shells that let us hear
> Sacred whispers are the key,
> To the history we hold dear.
>
> Stone People we will hear you.
> Teach us the ancient ways,
> So we may build a future
> Based on prayer and praise.

The Stone People are the record holders for the Earth Mother. These great teachers can give the seeker much knowledge regarding the history of our planet and her children. That is to say, the body of Mother Earth is made of rock that breaks and moves with weather, breaking down into smaller stones that later become soil. Rocks carry records and transport electromagnetic energy on Mother's surface. The Stone People collect the energy and hold it for later use. The mineral kingdom is dense matter that has a magnetic quality that allows the stones to record all that occurs on the planet.

Many healing uses are being discovered for various members of the Stone Clan. Native Americans have always used clear quartz crystals for focus and clarity. Medicine people in the northern part of Turtle Island have carved and carried many fetishes made of crystal for centuries. The magnification of knowledge and ability are assisted by using the clear quartz crystals.

Different types of coloured stone have been used throughout the centuries for healing purposes. These are usually specific minerals that can tell a healer of their gifts and talents in assisting a healing process.

The Stone People who are teachers of the children of Earth come in many forms. The stones used in traditional Native healing are those found by river banks, along canyon walls and washes, which come to the surface via natural erosion. There is nothing wrong with taking from the Earth Mother if something is given back to her. It is always a good idea to offer tobacco or to plant a tree in gratitude for that which was removed in another place.

The Stone People who come to the surface of our Earth are the record holders. Many will become soil in future generations due to erosion. These Stone People are considered common rocks by those not versed in the language of the stones. Every marking on a rock has a meaning and many times when intuition is used, faces of two-leggeds (humans) and creature beings can be seen on the surfaces of stones. These faces are the connections that stone has to the children of Earth.

Nothing is ever put on our paths without a reason.

When we are attracted to a certain rock and we pick that Stone Person up, it has a lesson for us. The language of the stones is a personal discovery with many messages for each individual. Since we are unique in our tastes, different Stone People will attract us.

Each Stone Person can be a protecting and guiding force in life. The Sioux Indians call their protection stones Wo-Ties and the Seneca call them Teaching Stones. In Seneca tradition, any stone with a natural hole through it will bring protection to the holder. Stones have been used by Native medicine people for divination purposes for centuries. In some tribes they use the stones to forecast the future recipient of the ceremony. Stones can also be used to assist in finding missing items or persons. Although women are participants in these ceremonies, traditionally all Yuwipi medicine is reserved for a special society of rock medicine men. These medicine men are growing more scarce as time passes. However the few that still remain are very gifted and highly revered among the Ogalala, Lakota and Dakota Sioux.

The role that Stone People play in the tribes of Native America varies from tribe to tribe. Each tribe has specific teachings that were passed to it through the stones over the past few centuries. Since these lessons were based on trial and error, which then becomes tradition, each medicine person has varying use for the stones. The Paiute medicine people knew how to use an extract from the poisonous stone cinnebar in small quantities to heal certain illnesses among the people. The Tonkawas used limestone with impressions of fossils to connect them to the ancestors. The Commanches used certain types of flint to make special arrowheads that were called medicine arrows and were used in healing ceremonies. The Apaches used certain coloured stones on a trail to divine the paths leading to the Sacred Mountains.

Each tradition has found separate uses for the language of the stones and has revered the teachings of the rock nation as being messages of the Earth Mother.

Every lesson on how to live in harmony on the Earth can be learned through connecting to the Stone People. The fact that each rock is a part of the body of our Mother speaks for itself. When we seek to slow down our minds and feel the earthing influence that brings balance and serenity, a Stone Person is our tool. When nervous habits run us ragged, we are not feeling connected to the Earth Mother. Sure signs of being off balance are overeating, talking too much, addictions, compulsions, or erratic behaviour. To calm the body, mind or spirit, we need only to hold a Stone Person and breathe until the nervousness passes.

This earthing influence is a way of anchoring the body to the Earth Mother and feeling the security of her nurturing influence. The impressions of every act of creation from the moment our planet cooled until the present are contained in the bodies of the Stone People. This great fount of wisdom is ours as a gift if we are willing to connect with the stone teachers. The calming effect we receive is the wisdom of these rock elders, who were the first historians for all our relations. Their mission is to be of service to the two-leggeds. Now it is up to us to seek and accept their gifts.

## Stone Application

The Stone People mark a time in which knowing will be revealed to you. Your personal records are held by these libraries of rock. Childhood memories may return and allow you to piece together a part of your personal puzzle. Memories of past lives or *déjà vu* could bring new awareness. Whatever the case, you are now in a position to know where you came from and where you are going.

A Stone Person can assist you in focusing your intent, dispelling confusion, changing habits, retrieving records from long ago or getting rounded. Allow these teachers to become your allies and discover a new world. Listen to the whispers of the mineral kingdom and your heart will know.

In all cases, the Stone People ask you to open your mind because new understanding is always there. The knowledge is based on Earth records and may change the way in which you view life. These ancient friends are the oldest children of Earth and only ask us to stop and listen.

## How Stones Have Been Used

We now know that the oldest rocks on Earth actually came from outer space in the form of meteorites. The stone type is called chondrite and the earliest pieces can be dated as 4,600 million years old. It wasn't until much later that the rocks began to form actually on the Earth – some 4,200 years ago, mere youngsters!

So who else cottoned on to how valuable they are?

Since the dawn of time, people have been drawn to the energies of the stones. You only have to look around to see the traces we have left from centuries of walking on Mother Earth. We have carried monstrous stones unspeakable distances, to honour kings and gods. The human race has created monuments of stone, and carved human faces and those of gods in the stones. Left behind are the reminders of mysterious or forgotten people, such as the statues on Easter Island, the Sphinx, the Pyramids, the Inca temples, Machu Picchu and Stonehenge. More recently in America, there is Mount Rushmore.

Lava stone and basalt stone were used for building altars for religious or magical practices. The Incas coated theirs in gold and constructed Sun and Moon temples for worship. I saw in 2000 with my own eyes on a visit to Peru just how revered this stone was. The phenomenal distances the Incas carried the stones, and the incredible sizes they worked with, were impossible to imagine. It was very evident in every religious, respected or valued place we saw that there were no lengths they wouldn't go to to build stone temples for worship.

There are the worry stones people carry in their pockets; and stone fetishes are created for many forms of healing, rebirth, wealth and relationships.

- As part of their deep respect for stones, Native Americans use heated stones in their sweat lodges, usually the bluish-to-black stones. They also use a Sun-heated (heliotherapy) stone on the belly of a woman when her menses are painful, to relieve the pain.

- In the Sioux tradition a boy going through manhood would lie on a hard rock and put smooth stones between his toes to teach him the difference between hard and soft, female and male, for a beginning of understanding how important it is to balance one's life. Maybe we could introduce this into primary school lesson plans!

- Many shamans, medicine people and spiritual healers from all over the world use stones and crystals in their healing ceremonies. Each colour and type of stone reflects an energy, purpose, clearing and releasing effect on the client as it is being used. Very few are chosen to learn from a spiritual teacher how to use the stones for healing. Usually a shaman will pass on the knowledge of healing to one special student before they pass into the light to rejoin their creator. This is one reason why there is very little out there for research purposes.

- The healing women of the Mapuche tribes in Chile used black stones in their healing work and for divination.

- In Hawaii the Kahunas use lava stones in their healing treatments, and they wrap the stone in a ki (ti) leaf. The lava stone represents healing and protection.

- In the Philippines it is a common practice to use a rough basalt stone that we know as pumice to slough off old and dry skin. Many women today still use these porous pumice stones in the bath to maintain smooth, silky skin. We know it as pumice and in fact it is the only type of stone that floats – remarkable, amazing and basalt!

- In Russia there is a tradition of using heated black stones in baths. People line the bottom of the bath-tub with hot stones and then lie down on the smooth stones, soaking in the soothing warm energy that radiates from each stone.

- In the days when cowboys were roaming the United States it was a common practice for them to heat stones in the fire and then place them on the ground under their bedding. The stones' heated energies kept them warm at night, and the stones were also more giving to the body than the earth for comfort. Watch with a keen eye next time you settle in for a good old black and white Western.

- The Japanese people use the smooth black stones to keep their abdomens warm after a meal. It is customary for them not to eat a lot at one time, and this is achieved by placing two or three warm stones in the sash that is wrapped around their waist. This gives them a sense of being fuller for a longer period of time. One might even be able to claim that LaStone can be used for weight loss.
- The Maya Indians use a divination stone to tell them what illness a patient has, and what the treatment(s) should be to aid the person back to good health. This is very similar to the use of a crystal ball.
- In China the use of heated stones to relieve tired muscles dates back to before the Shang Dynasty (c. 2000–1500 BC).

And here is Mary's story about her treatment and the use of the Stone Clan People.

Lava stones are a reminder of creation, the beginning of time, when Mother Earth was covered with water. As new life breathed into her, her body erupted from the depths of her soul and brought forth the land, a place where new forms of life would thrive and evolve. The eruption of the volcanoes reaching to Father Sun brought forth the land, which we as humans now claim to own – a place where air-breathing creatures could crawl out of the waters of their Mother Earth and evolve into new forms.

In time, the two-legged creatures began to spread, honouring Mother Earth and Father Sun as their givers of life, accepting their place in the chain of life and living by the rules of nature. As time passed we, the two-legged beings, began to spread and rule over the other clans. Then came the time when men needed to rule each other. Soon the connections to Mother Earth and Father Sun were no longer respected; we created new gods in many forms, always trying to create what we always had in the beginning, not realising we had never lost it.

Some cultures teach that the Stone Clan People (stones, rocks, boulders), have the memories of all the events on this planet, if not the universe. They agree to aid each human in their own personal journeying of healing and transformation by enhancing our memories and allowing us to view life in a more balanced and spiritual way. We only have to look within our soul to truly know the answers to all our questions. By using the stones in a body treatment we are again honouring the powers of Mother Earth, allowing her children to join together for a deeper understanding of the order of life.

There is very little written down about the use of stones as treatment for people for any reason. Most, if not all, treatments that use stones are passed down from one healer or medicine person to the next. It is an honour to be chosen to learn the art of healing through the energies of Mother Earth and her children, the Stone Clan People.

## CHAPTER SIX

# Types of Stone Used

WE HAVE STONES for the neck, the toes, the face, the tummy, the spine, the chakras and much, much more.

## Basalt Stones for Heat

Nothing is left to chance – even the number 54 is auspicious as the 5 plus 4 add up to 9, which is a very important number in therapy. The entire treatment is subject to knowledge, training, wisdom and intuition – Oh! and 54 stones.

We use 54 carefully chosen basalt stones in LaStone Therapy. Each stone has a specific purpose and excepting 5 stones, all of them are exactly paired. A massage therapist uses both hands for most strokes. This can also be done in LaStone Therapy, but using similar stones in each hand, and thus making the strokes feel balanced and even. This is no mean feat and another example of how perfect this treatment can be.

LaStone Therapy uses basalt pebbles for the treatment. In order to know why this stone was chosen, Mary Nelson asked a friend, Bill Updegrove, who works in the US Geological Survey at the University of Arizona, for assistance. Bill was very helpful, and he and his colleagues agreed to research the stone and give a breakdown of what they found. Chemical, mineralogical and geological questions were asked. They used a variety of methods of analysis: mass spectrometry, X-ray fluorescence, X-ray diffraction, thin-section analysis, and lengthy debates that did not always end in agreement.

Listening to the results of all the research they shared, Mary began to realise that basalt was and is in fact one of the most common stones on the planet, and one of the simplest.

The geologists and mineralogists found that the stones were made up of orthoclase, pyroxene, plagioclase feldspar and vitrified silicates; augite, iron and magnesium constituents were also found.

The type of basalt that is used in La Stone Therapy is modified igneous rock that is formed by volcanic and sedimentary action. When rocks of the Earth's crust and upper mantle melt, they form magma, which is expelled by volcanic activity – eruption. When we see this happen on television or more close at hand (if we happen to be in a safe place to view a volcanic eruption!) then we see that these stones are truly thrown up out of Mother Earth. The hugely energetic force spews out materials that eventually become the stones that will be used on your body during a treatment. That thought alone is pretty amazing.

The most common material erupted is basalt. This is the most abundant of the volcanic rocks, especially plentiful in those regions that have undergone volcanic disturbance within geologically recent times. Basalt forms from the more fluid types of lava as it cools and hardens. It actually forms the ocean floor that covers 68 per cent of the world's surface area.

Most present-day volcanoes erupt basaltic material. This type of basalt is usually made up of polycrystalline olivine, an iron-magnesium silicate. There are several varieties of basalt. Most contain olivine and iron-magnesium silicate, and those containing notable quantities of this mineral are known as olivine basalt.

Olivine basalt is a fine-grained, black stone that is very dense and forms fine crystalline masses. The density of the stones is 2.5 times the weight per volume of water. The hardness is 7 on the Mohs' Scale of 1–10, a diamond being a 10. This basalt has typically been formed downwind of a volcano, that is to say it has cooled slowly. The rocks have changed their composition as metamorphosis has taken place, and have crystallised again and again; this is the cause of their great density and variety of colour, from black to purple, grey to dark green. They have also been broken and eroded by steam or water activity.

The huge pieces of rock have then been washed along a river bottom or across the seashore until eventually, some millions of years later, they have ended up as the extremely smooth, potato-shaped and sized pebbles that we use in the treatment. Basalt is dense and dark and by the time we see it, it is very smooth. It is also a type of stone clearly suited to being heated and to holding its heat for long periods of time.

Just as crystals are imbued with energetic and healing qualities, so is basalt. Energetically it is reputed to have some amazing properties as well. Basalt is said to provide you with the strength to continue through difficult times and can produce solidarity. It can help to diffuse anger and with providing understanding and guidance in situations that we need to recover from. It will help you through change while providing a stable 'rock' in life. It will help you diminish the negativity of your personality and enhance the positive side of yourself. It can be used to promote the health of the reproductive organs and systems, to enhance fertility and to develop personal physical strength. It can be recharged during both full and new Moons.

Basalt is also said to vibrate to the number 1 and to represent the astrological signs of Taurus and Cancer, signs of strength and stability. So not only does basalt work on the physical level by being able to deliver a slow, constant release of heat, but it also works energetically to result in a total body, mind and spirit experience.

# Marble Stones for Cooling

There are 27 marble stones in most of the sets used in LaStone Therapy – I say most as we source these sets from many places around the world and sometimes they vary, but normally 27 is the number. If you think about it, 2 plus 7 equals 9 ... just another example of the details in this treatment.

The marble is made for us; you very rarely find marble in pebble form as it would simply break up if tumbled on a shoreline or river bed. Each shape is carefully designed to do the most important work and to fit neatly into the therapist's hand, in order to be able to switch from hot to cool in moments.

Like basalt, marble has been on a long and historic journey before it reaches our treatment rooms. Thinking about this just for a moment is a great appreciation of how Mother Nature provides everything we need.

Marble is a metamorphosed limestone. In fact the term marble is used for a variety of rocks. Marble in its raw form is coarsely crystalline. When limestone is exposed to very high temperatures, new crystals of calcite grow and form the compact rock we know as marble. In contrast to basalt, marble is very soft and easy to break or scratch.

Limestone is a sedimentary rock that consists of the remains of once-living organisms. In some examples we can clearly see the animals in the rock itself. Limestone is constantly being formed in the collecting sediments on the sea floor. It is the most common sedimentary rock on Earth. Salt water covers nearly 75 per cent of the Earth's surface. So if basalt makes up 68 per cent of the ocean floor, then we can start to see that limestone, i.e. marble, is formed on top of basalt.

Limestone also harbours the largest reservoir of carbon at or near the surface of the Earth. Calcium carbonate ($CaCO_3$) is the main component of limestone and it comes from lime-secreting organisms, some of which are algaes. Together with coral-forming plants and animals, these algaes create limestone reefs.

Much of the fossil record on Earth is contained in limestone, and its study has contributed to our knowledge of the evolution of life and Earth's history.

Eventually, the depth of these gathering sediments increases to the point where they become stabilised and cemented together. The weight of the sea water and loose sediment above helps to press the layers into the sedimentary rock, in this case limestone. The layers of limestone then become bonded to the ocean floor, the continent. The continent rests on the crystal plates of the Earth. The crust of the Earth is some twenty miles below the continents and six miles or so below the oceans. The crystal plates drift around on the 1,800-mile-thick mantle, which in turn floats on an extremely hot liquid core like dumplings on a stew. It is the interaction of the crust, the mantle and the core that turns our relatively soft sedimentary limestone into an extremely hard, metamorphic marble.

The word metamorphosise means 'to change form', like a cocoon changes into a butterfly. In geology, metamorphism occurs deep in the crust of the Earth. As the crystal plates slide around, they run into each other. Often, a product of these collisions is a fault zone, where earthquakes tend to occur due to the release of pressure building between the plates. At other times one plate will subduct, or slide under, another plate. When a subduction occurs, the sinking plate is driven deep under the crust. As this plate gets deeper, it is subjected to the immense heat that is rising up from the liquid core. Earth core temperatures are thousands of degrees high.

Under these conditions the sinking plate of sediment is subject not only to increasing pressure, but also to extreme temperatures that melt the sediment. The sedimentary limestone layers become liquid or semi liquid, like glass, and can stay in this state for hundreds of thousands, even millions, of years. The subducted plate eventually makes it to the surface again, and when it does it starts to cool and congeal and becomes solid. The rate at which the rock cools determines what form and composition the new metamorphic layers will take. These rates of cooling vary immensely throughout the vastness of the rising plate.

In order for limestone to transform into marble, the limestone has to be pure calcium carbonate – over 90 per cent. The rate of cooling and the pounds of pressure need to be very consistent over hundreds or even thousands of years as the liquid limestone cools and grows marble crystals through the process of precipitation. If the factors for creating marble are not present, minerals like chalk, talc and calcite form. These minerals can be adjacent to each other or form in isolated pockets throughout the continent.

The continents of the Earth are always on the move, drifting wherever the factors deep below them dictate. Before our present-day arrangement of continents, the marble rock may have already been forming for 200 to 300 million years. As the continents and plates emerged and rearranged to form the present-day continents, these metamorphic rocks and their pockets of marble were thrust up to form mountain ranges. As these mountain ranges were eroded by thousands of years of weather, some pockets of marble became accessible to our mining tools.

Marble was formed on Earth via the entire geological process – a process that continues to create marble even as you read this. Marble, holding immense periods of time and records of the evolution of life, bears intrinsic beauty in its crystals. Marble, when driven to the surface of the land and subjected to the factors of erosion, becomes the sands of rivers and may someday come to rest at the bottom of the ocean, tainting the formation of limestone. The cycle is never ending.

Energetically, marble is reported to have phenomenal properties almost as stunning as the process of its physical formation. It is used to provide clarity and to enable deeper meditation and suspended states. It promotes peak states of meditation and total recall of dreams.

Marble helps to activate the unused portions of the mind, strength and self-control, the power of thought and the peace of serenity. It helps to promote purification and thought control and processing, enabling us to actualise our true wishes and desires.

Spiritually, marble transforms unhappy circumstances. It helps to change dynamically things we thought we had to put up with. Emotionally, marble brings any repressed contents of our consciousness to the surface. It helps us to rid ourselves of emotional dissatisfaction. Mentally, marble opens up new perspectives and stimulates creative solutions to problems that we previously could not see a way out of.

Physically, marble improves the processing of calcium in the body. It stimulates the metabolism, fortifies immunity and encourages the healing of tissue and bone. It also regulates and strengthens the heart.

Marble can promote nurturing instincts and help with common sense practice in affairs of the heart, home and appetite. It is a stone to 'provide protection', both physically and emotionally. It brings balance to physical and worldly matters.

Marble assists in the aspects of patience and determination during participation in body-fitness programmes, and has long been used in homeopathy and naturopathy. It has also been said that ruin marble – marble from ancient ruins – can aid in connection with ancient civilisations and sharing the goals of ancient cultures. The stone vibrates with the number 6 and again is associated with the astrological sign of Cancer.

There are numerous different types of stone on this Earth. LaStone Therapy chose basalt and marble. Their very specific origins and properties make the treatment so perfect.

The stones deliver a deeply healing treatment through use of the optimum temperature and mineral combination. They are naturally attuned to bring balance and healing on every level.

# Colour, Shape and Size

A note from Mary Nelson:

Basalt comes in many colours. Dark grey, green and black stay hottest the longest. Therefore any of these three colours will work for the hot stone massage of LaStone Therapy. Some of the dark reds/purples will also stay hot. It is believed by some cultures around the world that the colour black represents male energies and the colour white represents female energies. Some colours are associated with the chakras.

I have found over the years that using black/purple and greenish basalt stones for the heated part and shades of white marble for the cooled part of LaStone Therapy brings balance and grounding to the therapy, for myself and my clients – not to mention the fact that it is just plain fun, having the contrast of the light and dark working with me in aiding my clients on a path of healing.

During many years of working with the basalt stones I have found them very hard to find, in just the right size and shape to do the work. The correct texture and density of the stones is very important in maintaining the temperature needed to do LaStone Therapy. The stones that are needed to do the deep-tissue work, the belly, sacrum and scapula/rhomboid work, seem to be the hardest to find.

One can look for years before finding the exact size and shape. At present we have been blessed with AML LaStone and Stone People to do the hunting and harvesting for us. AML LaStone and Stone People have taken great pains to ensure the stones will indeed hold the heat needed in order to effectively perform LaStone Therapy.

Mother Earth supplies us with a beautiful stone, tumbled naturally in the belly of her rivers. If you have received treatments from stones supplied by LaStone-approved people, or received your stones for practice from LaStone-recognised suppliers, you have now experienced a set of stones that not only will maintain the temperature you need, but will also feel lovely in your hands and on the body. A natural set of stones is wonderful to work with, and you will have every stone you need to do the heated part of LaStone Therapy.

As for marble stones, there are no such things in the natural world. That leaves us in the skilled hands of an artist. We have been blessed with a few such people who are willing to hand-make marble stones for us to use in LaStone Therapy. The marble stones are cut and hand-sanded to just the right size and shape needed to assist us in the bodywork that cryotherapy was meant to do for humans – bringing down inflammation and starting the healing process.

If you choose to order a set of marble stones from LaStone suppliers, you will see the beauty in each stone as you begin to experience the excitement you will feel as you incorporate ener-gies of both black and white, hot and cold in your treatments. Give thanks to Mother Earth, the Stone Clan People and all that exist, for each of your clients will know the blessings that they have received because you brought them closer to their own creation.

## The Stones Are Alive

You may be starting to realise that the stones we use in LaStone Therapy take on a life of their own, and that the therapist just adds some assistance, intuition and guidance to the treatment. In this connection, the article below is an interesting and modern interpretation of what the Native Americans have known and tried to tell us all along. Written by Rabbi Lionel Blue and published in the *Times* on 5 August, 1996, the article is entitled 'In a sense, even the rocks breathe'.

There is too much of a distinction made between the conscious-ness of people and of animals and of inanimate things. I don't think there is a cast iron distinction between live and dead matter, or at least the distinction is of degree, not of kind – there might be consciousness in a lump of rock. We concentrate on our own consciousness, but humanity will disappear before it understands even the consciousness of a gnat.

Even rocks breathe in a strange sort of way. It might well be our parochialism that leads us to think that we are so enormously different, that we have nothing in common with other things. Certainly we are a very distinguished lot, but there may be others to whom our consciousness is of no more significance than that of rock to us.

If you ask what is the purpose of the universe, it is a matter of moving into consciousness. Whether that movement will be evolution or explosion, I don't know. A rock may be farther back than us, but it is part of this movement and will explode into consciousness itself.

This way of thinking would not sound radical in Eastern thought, where a continuum is acknowledged, where we and all other things are part of a bigger play. But we are interested only in the little bit of the universe that we know: we will never know how a beetle looks at us, or at the world. *As soon as you get away from an idea of humans at the centre, you have a different view of everything.*

Matter is only one stage of a journey to consciousness, which is the only part of the journey that I can discern – there must be other states, beyond anything I can possibly know. That is why we feel a frisson when we hear a line of poetry.

And that frisson cannot be explained by electrical activity in the brain. There is electrical activity in a rock! A rock has something going on too!

There are many levels of consciousness and we can't make these very firm classifications from our human standpoint, because from the standpoint of another form of consciousness we are the same as rocks.

Reality can be explained in so many ways that do not exclude each other. Science has been the glory of our time but it does not, alone, explain.

Science can describe consciousness or reality, and use its information – but you would also need some glint of a hunch, or a spark from another level, to get the whole thing going.

## CHAPTER SEVEN

# Obtaining and Using Stones

NOWADAYS THE STONES USED for LaStone can be supplied by approved suppliers for LaStone, but this wasn't always the case. Indeed, the people that harvest the stones for supply to LaStone therapists must go out and harvest in the way Mary describes below in detail. To simply take from the Earth would be to steal and certainly wouldn't drive the positive energy that is intrinsic to this treatment.

## Harvesting and Caring for the Stones

The choice of stone and respect for Mother Earth is crucial to a successful set of stones for practice. A set of stones supplied by a recognised company will make the treatment streamlined, flowing and perfect. Simply using a selection of randomly taken stones would certainly not do the job. The crucial element of honour is present in harvesting and maintaining the stones, and in return the stones will honour the treatment. From Mary:

Many tools and quite a bit of equipment are used for a LaStone treatment, but the most important is having the right set of stones – the true natural tools for the job. May you remember to thank Mother Earth for her gifts you have received.

At present, one must go out into the world to harvest basalt stones that are needed in the heated part of LaStone Therapy. The black-to-grey stones' qualities are stillness, sleep, rest, solidity, and little or no movement. They open energy channels and are for grounding and focusing. There is also a clear focus on the physical plane, a calming of the mind and a consecutive slowing of physical movement. This type of basalt stays hot longer than any other colour of the river rocks. I suggest that you find the stones you want to use in the general area of where you live. This way the electromagnetic energy of the stones and the people will be similar.

You can't go out and find the marble stones for the cold application of LaStone Therapy; they have to be hand-cut and hand-sanded.

Once you've obtained your stones for use in the heated treatments and in the cold application of LaStone Therapy, you may want to consider placing them on the ground outside every day for a period of three full Moons. This way their electromagnetic energy will adjust to the area of Mother Earth that you are living on. As we travel on Mother Earth the magnetic pull changes, and so do we and all of Earth's clan energies change and adjust to Mother Earth and the way that all things interact in the universe. You have experienced this when you have gone on holiday or moved – something seemed out of balance and it took you a few weeks to adjust to your new environment.

By placing the Stone Clan People on the ground every night for three full Moons, you will be allowing the stones to become one with the vibrations of Mother Earth. This too will work for you as you travel to different locations on her body. Take time to lie down on her surface, breathing in her heartbeat and feeling the energy exchange between you and your Mother, the Earth.

When looking for stones, look for the colour dark grey to black, even dark green, dark purple and some dark red. The smoother and glassier the stone, the longer it will stay hot when heated in water. You may have to wet the stone to see if it is what you are looking for. Keep in mind the shape of the stones needed for the treatment.

Collecting stones is not just a matter of picking up what you think will suit the purpose. Your intention must be to replenish the Earth and not to just take from it. There are a few steps to take to ensure that the man from the National Trust doesn't (quite rightly) tell you to put them back. This is how Mary goes about harvesting her stones.

Harvesting basalt stones from Mother Earth can be done in many ways. One only has to search one's spirit to know that it is important to give back to the Earth whenever you take from her. If we do not give back to Mother Earth when she supplies us with gifts, where does that leave the energy of the gift? There are many ways in which to thank Mother Earth for her gifts. You may read about these ceremonies in most books on crystals and stone healing, as well as in books on shamanism.

I would like to share with you one of the ways I choose to give back to Mother Earth when harvesting Stone Clan People. I always carry with me a pouch of bird seed, food for the birds as well as for the small creatures that roam the Earth. I verbally thank Spirit and Mother Earth for showing me her Stone Clan People. Over the past couple of years, I have learned to listen to the stones as they call out to me, and to know which ones want to come with me. These are the stones that carry the frequencies that will aid humans in reprogramming their memories and accessing their awareness of who they are as children of the light.

Before I begin a day's harvest, I cast the bird seed to Mother Earth, honouring each of the four directions, Above, Below, Within, Without and All Around. While doing so I give thanks for the seed and all that the Earth offers; the water, earth, plants, animals, and Stone Clan People. I ask her to show my feet the way to walk, my ears to hear and my heart to know how to find the stones for each one of us, so that we may all follow a path of self-healing.

Each stone has its own purpose in life. The colours correspond with those of the chakras in the body. For the use of heat I use the greyish/black basalt stones; this is, of course, what was channelled to me to use. As time goes by I continue to learn that on every continent all over Mother Earth, many shamans and medicine people have been chosen by these stones to do healing work for the humans on this planet. If you choose to use the greyish/black stones in your in LaStone Therapy, they represent yang/male, energy. The colour black helps to open energy channels by grounding and focusing the client's energy, and calming the mind and emotions, with a firm focus on the physical plane.

To balance our body-mind-spirit we must use both yin and yang. If the black stones are yang, then the white marble stones will compliment the male (black) stones with yin/female energy, the soft side of our Spirit. The white marble stone that has been chosen to be used in LaStone Therapy is softer than the basalt, and will stay colder longer and bring a great deal of contrast to the treatment. I find a great deal of excitement in using the two dramatic colours together. The colour white helps to heighten your awareness of who you are in this vast universe, opening your crown chakra to receiving information, and allowing you to walk in the light of your own Spirit.

Beyond the colours, the shapes have both yin and yang energies as well. The round stones are represented by the female/yin side of the universe. The oblong stones are in turn transferring the male/yang side of the spectrum. These colours, black or white, mixed with the shapes, round or oblong, will also aid in the delicate balance of bringing your body, mind and soul to perfect harmony. This energy exchange between the black/round stones or the white/oblong stones aids the client in a simple balance of both yin and yang. What a gift to give your clients, a gift of wholeness.

Once I get the stones home, I clean them and sort them, finding partners for each of them to be used together in a treatment. I keep the stones outdoors, some in sets ready for use in LaStone Therapy, some in groups of similar size and shape awaiting their time of use.

Mary Nelson wrote this note when she was explaining how she went about harvesting her own stones and then latterly when recognised companies started to harvest for therapists wishing to learn LaStone Therapy. The LaStone treatment has now become extremely busy and as such there are many companies supplying the stones but still following the very particular and strict criteria that keep the standards so high.

Simply owning stones is not enough. As soon as we start to use them in treatments they become the tools of our trade and as such we must take great care of them to ensure that they do the best they can. Just as we get tired at the end of a working day, the stones will also get tired. Just as we want to get out in the daylight if we have been in a beautifully lit room inside all day – so do the stones. If we do not recharge or energise our stones on a regular basis they will lose their own energy and the treatment will become soulless. You may still be wondering why, if the stones are inanimate objects, do they get tired? Well, they are not dead; they have a flow of natural energy even if you only believe they have molecules. These molecules need refreshments. From Mary:

I wash my stones at the end of every day of treatments. Once the stones have dried, I place them in a bed of salts, using Epsom salts or sea salt. Don't use commercial table salt, which often contains aluminum. Salt helps to clear and recharge the stones for the next day's work. You may also lay them out in the form of a medicine wheel on the massage table or outside on Mother Earth, as they love this form of energy work. As often as possible, I place my stones in the Sun and Moon's light for recharging. Stones have energy, or frequencies, just as all substances have. The use of salts, Sun, Moon and water helps to bring back the energy lost when they are doing their work on clients.

I cannot emphasise this enough: you must clean and store your stones daily. If you don't give thanks for what the stones have done for you during the day, they will lose their energies. This is a fact. You can look at it as electromagnetic energy or you can open your heart and see it as I do. The stones do an enormous amount of healing for us during our work. They not only balance, ground and aid in healing our clients; they also heal our hands, thumbs and wrists.

Without taking time for ceremonies for the stones on a daily basis, they will lose their inner energies. They will not stay hot/cold for you during your work. You will begin to wonder why your roaster isn't keeping the stones hot any longer. You will begin to raise the thermostat, thinking something is wrong, and not realising that all you need to do is get the stones outside in their element. The stones love to be outside in water or lying on the Earth.

A word of caution: if you are lucky enough to get your stones outside during an electrical storm, beware, for the stones will just soak up the energies and will be much hotter than usual for the next treatments. My clients always comment on how hot the stones are after a storm, even though I don't change the setting on the roaster. The stones are energised; they love to be outside during a storm, or a full Moon. The marble is energised in the same way. Clients don't seem to mind the increase in the cold, for if you use the cold stones on areas of inflammation, as you should, then the extra cold is welcomed and soaked into the body for healing purposes.

I invite you to challenge this belief of mine and see if your stones don't lose their lustrous appearance and ability to hold in heat and cold. You and your stones will become tired, and will not be excited about your work together. You will have to exchange stones more often due to the fact that there isn't enough heat in one stone to do the work you want to accomplish. The cold stones will begin to feel sticky and lifeless. The spirit of the stones will have slipped away somewhere and your clients will no longer comment on how incredible the treatment is with the stones.

At this point I pray that you remember my words and take all your stones (every stone or crystal you own) outside and give thanks for their time and the energies that they are so willing to share with you. It will be then and only then that the life of the stones will come back to you in your work. The excitement of collecting your stones from outside the next morning will be that of getting a new puppy or opening up a special present. You will have been energised as well as the stones, and all will work happily together once more. Only if you can believe in this connection with the stones and Mother Earth will you prosper in your business. So open your heart to the healing powers within the stones and you and your clients will soar further than your dreams have taken you so far.

I completely understand that sometimes it is difficult to 'believe' all aspects of LaStone Therapy, and I was that way inclined when I first began. Indeed, I did take up Mary's invitation to challenge her belief, with interesting but predictable results.

I used my stones and then washed them at the end of the day and put them away until next time. Some time later I noticed that during treatments my water tank was still reading as 57 degrees centigrade but the stones didn't feel very hot in my hands. I decided the thermostat had broken. I bought a new thermometer and tested the tank. The temperature reading was correct, but still the stones felt lukewarm.

Then I remembered the information on recharging. I decided to take my stones home and put them out overnight. Sure enough, and actually to my great amusement, the stones proved the theory right. Next day they were at full heat and power, yet the water-heater dial had remained unchanged. They were back in business after just one night out.

These are the techniques we practitioners have to utilise to make sure we keep the stones happy and working hard.

## Taking Special Care of the Stones

As mentioned, taking care of your work-tools is as essential to therapists for maintaining standards as it is for any craftsman or manual worker. The saying that a good workman never blames his tools is very appropriate here. If the therapist does not take care of their stones it will be totally their fault if the treatment deteriorates and moves from being a total mind-body-spirit experience to simply a rub with some warm stones.

I have mentioned ways of recharging the stones; there are crystals that we can use to enhance this 'taking care', and some other processes that we can go through to ensure that the stones are at their best at all times.

### More on recharging the stones

We use labradorite crystal to recharge basalt stones and can also use moonstone to recharge the marble stones – although labradorite will do the job for both quite adequately. We can also use natural salt and the energy of the Moon and Sun to recharge the stones. In addition, mandalas or medicine wheels can serve the stones on a more regular basis.

Perhaps the most powerful way to recharge both the basalt and the marble stones is to get them out into the natural elements, to where they come from, or 'home'. If we have spent all day inside working, we want to go outside to get some fresh air. If we have been away for a while we want to go home and so do the stones. They can recharge with Earth energy and resonate with familiar surroundings. Better still is to get them outside during the full Sun or full Moon – the most invigorating and most creative times of the natural Earth.

Obviously, this is not practical to do every day, not least because of the weight of the stones and the logistics of getting them in and out of work every day. This is more a monthly process.

In the meantime, we can recharge the stones by putting them in a mandala or medicine wheel on the massage couch or plinth, or in a space in the treatment area. Creating a mandala is a way of honouring flow and energy, and leaving the stones in some form of pattern or design will help them to recharge. It is nice to scatter the pattern with natural sea salt, which is cleansing and balancing, and we also know that salt was an extremely rare and valuable substance in years gone by. Alternatively, we can use natural or wild sage with the stones as this is an extremely cleansing plant used in many Native American rituals.

Many cultures use mandalas, or circles, to represent the total circle of life and birth and the ceaseless spinning to death, which gives rise to birth, which is followed by death and so on. The 'circle of life' and 'this mortal coil' are phrases that show how we think of life as either a visual or actual circle or sphere.

Native Americans use mandalas to represent the wheel of life. The Native American mandala is also called a medicine wheel. This wheel is marked out into the compass points: north, south, east and west; the four seasons: spring, summer, autumn and winter; and the four elements: water, earth, air and fire.

It seems that whatever your belief, you can use the imagery of the circle and the power of nature to create your own personal mandala. You are able to focus on your own life, your own beliefs and your own path to achieve whatever you wish to achieve. It is the same for the stones – reflection and regeneration.

Placing a piece of either labradorite (or spectralite) or moonstone with their stones – labradorite with basalt and moonstone with marble – ensures that the stones remain neutral and cleansed both during and in between treatments.

## *Labradorite*

Labradorite is a beautiful dark crystal with blue or green flashes of iridescent colour.

- Spiritually, this crystal helps us to see our goals and intentions. Labradorite helps us with tuning in to our own intuition.
- Emotionally, labradorite brings up forgotten memory and gives us depth of feeling. It stimulates our imagination and makes us contemplative and introspective.
- Mentally, labradorite helps us to develop a child-like enthusiasm, and many, many new ideas. It makes us more creative.
- Physically, labradorite alleviates colds, flu, rheumatic illness and gout. It is also calming and can help to lower blood pressure.
- Essentially, labradorite is a crystal for wisdom. It is a protective stone, and deflects unwanted energies from the aura and prevents energy leakage. It aligns physical and etheric bodies, raises consciousness and grounds spiritual energy into the body. It synthesises intellectual thought with intuitive wisdom, and accesses spiritual purpose. It also regulates the metabolism, gives us insight without searching and protects our aura during meditation or energy work – as does fluorite.

## *Moonstone*

We use moonstone to charge the marble stones as it is a female stone to the masculine labradorite. As its name suggests, it is aligned to the Moon and is therefore associated with intuition, fertility and the heart.

- Spiritually, moonstone encourages medium abilities and dreams.
- Emotionally, moonstone refines our perception and intuition. It allows the memory of dreams, helps to diffuse anger and balances emotional over-reaction.

- Mentally, moonstone opens us to sudden or irrational impulses. It encourages serendipity.
- Physically, moonstone balances hormonal production and nature's rhythms within the body. It can enhance fertility and help with menstrual problems, both during and after childbirth. It can also calm digestion and be fabulously detoxifying.

## Wild or white sage

This herbal plant is used in Native American traditions in a cleansing ritual. The burning of the sage in an area or over an object represents a clearing of negativity and a neutralising effect on the environment. Native American shamans use plants, animals and other natural objects as helpers or guardians in their work. In LaStone Therapy, we use sage to protect and cleanse.

There really is no excuse not to look after your stones, and the ritual used for doing so is just as powerful for the therapist as it is for the stones.

We give all students of LaStone detailed instructions on how to ensure that they make the best of their stones. Below is a copy of a note that we give to therapists to reinforce the message about looking after the tools of their trade. As you can see, all the techniques Mary talked about, and the added knowledge of crystal usage and Native American beliefs about sage as a cleansing and neutralising plant, are included.

---

### A Note to Therapists – Ways to Recharge and Energise the Stones

There are many ways to recharge or energise your stones. If you do not do this your stones will misbehave. Take care of them and they will take care of you. If your stones are not staying hot or will not heat up despite your heater showing a true reading, they are telling you that they need a bit of TLC!

These are the ways to achieve this.

Make sure you wash the stones every time you have finished with them, and give them fresh water every day you use them. Don't stew them in old, dirty water overnight, and don't put them in the dishwasher. If they are sticky, washing them in hot, soapy water or wiping them with surgical spirit is the quickest way to get the oil off. But every day that you use them, or if you haven't used them for a while and are preparing for treatments, you must do one of the following:

- Use labradorite for recharging basalt, moonstone for recharging marble.
- Or leave the stones out in the full Moon every month.
- Or get them out in the Sun.
- Or put them on the earth in a medicine wheel.
- Or leave them in your room in a medicine wheel.
- Or store them with natural sea salt sprinkled on them.
- Or smudge them by passing burning white sage over them for cleansing.

By taking these basic steps you will ensure that you will get the most out of the stones for every treatment.

As therapists, we should do something to cleanse and recharge ourselves each day as well. We should embody everything we wish for our clients – we need to be healthy, balanced and energised. Make sure you recharge yourself each day, as well as the stones. If you don't you may well confuse the stones about who they should treat, the client or the therapist. Don't confuse them; care for them.

And now for the science.

# Thermotherapy – Using Heat and Cold

Now that we know about the stones and how to care for and maintain them, we can look at why we heat and cool them. Why isn't the combination of their energy and their properties enough? Adding thermotherapy to the power of the natural energy of the stones makes you realise just how much power and how many layers the treatment has.

The use of hot and cold temperatures within the same treatment is extremely beneficial, if not crucial. When we talk about the application of hot and cold temperatures during a treatment we are looking at the initial short-term applications. If we keep to short-term applications the body is able to work at optimum levels, and the application of the therapist of hot and cold in the correct amounts, and for the correct amount of time, enables the body to concentrate on cleansing, rejuvenation and repair. If we use the temperatures for too long, the body needs to stop the 'repair' process and move in to protect and survive. Getting the balance of application right is essential.

Bathing in hot water is simply wonderful. Getting into a warm bath and relaxing for a while can do no end of good. Snuggling under a duvet on a cool night can relax and indulge. Now, imagine being in a hot bath and instead of the water slowly cooling and then you getting out of the bath when you have had enough, you are asked to stay in the water and it is kept at the temperature it was when you started – nice and hot. Pretty soon you might begin to feel a bit too hot, as if you are overheating, or you may even feel a bit faint and in need of some air, or at least cooling of some sort. This doesn't make the relaxing bath seem nice any more; in fact it sounds quite claustrophobic.

In the same way, imagine waking in the middle of the night and feeling far too hot. The once-comforting duvet has now become an overheating machine, and you immediately kick it off or stick an arm or a leg out of the bed to cool down. Imagine the same scenario again, but with you waking and finding yourself too hot. You are unable to throw the covers off or stick a limb out of bed; you have to stay where you are, all tucked in. You will experience the same feelings of overheating and fainting. Your body cannot tolerate such temperatures for this period of time. Once it feels too warm it will attempt to cool down. It will send blood away from its centre and out to the extremities, so that it cools down and doesn't 'cook' our internal organs. Long-term application of heat will cause the body to go into protection mode – not very relaxing or therapeutic.

These are the effects of the short- and long-term applications of heat: incredibly relaxing and therapeutic in the short term (and we will go on to see just how incredible the effects can be) to uncomfortable and depleting in the longer term.

In the same way, short-term application of cold can be wonderfully refreshing, but longer term application becomes freezing and debilitating. You go outside on a hot day to feel the cool, refreshing breeze on your face and arms. You cool down and feel balanced again. Now think how you would begin to feel if you were still sitting in that breeze a few minutes later. Your arms get goose pimples and you begin to shiver; you have become too cold and your body doesn't like it any more. The body needs to protect itself from freezing. Just as with the over-heating, your body will take blood to the core organs to protect them and prevent them from cooling down to a dangerous and stagnating level.

It soon becomes clear that we need to make sure our LaStone Therapy treatments observe the correct balance and application of hot and cold. A treatment should achieve the optimum benefit of alternating temperatures and all the effects these have, without any of the negative 'protect and survive' mechanisms being bought into play by the body itself. With a little knowledge, some wisdom and a lot of intuition, the LaStone therapist will get this balance perfect for every treatment.

The basic effects of short-term applications of hot and cold are given below. The beneficial effects are quite phenomenal and totally underestimated by most of us – no longer will a cold shower be a bad thing!

Here comes the science.

## Heat

The short-term effect of heat on the body is fabulously thera-peutic. When we talk about short term we are looking at anything between five and fifteen minutes. It is entirely depend-ent on the individual, their current health and their body's tolerance to heat. There are some people who can tolerate the hottest summer's day that the Sun can throw at them, yet there are others who need to retire to the shade and the cool breezes after five minutes. Observing a fifteen-minute maximum ensures that the body is perfectly happy with the temperature while defi-nitely benefitting from the therapeutic effects.

It is no coincidence that when we are ill, we have a tempera-ture. Although this is not short term, it does show that 'hot housing' the body will create an environment for the body in which it will be able to fight illness, process germs, build immu-nity and get better sooner. Fever is the body's way of applying thermotherapy – hot and cold in alternate application. Fever gives us periods of sweating and periods of shivers. This creates the optimum environment for the body to process illness and recover. Hydrotherapy is the external application of thermother-apy through the use of water.

### Application of heat:

• **Causes vasodilation** This is a widening of the blood vessels which in turn increases the blood flow around the body. Imagine that the blood is the fuel for the body, the petrol that keeps the body functioning at total efficiency. Increasing the blood flow and enabling the blood to pump more efficiently will ensure that the whole body will benefit immediately and totally. Waste products will be flushed out and internal organs cleansed. Everything will be boosted and on 'full flow'.

- **Increases circulation** If we have increased the blood flow around the body then we have definitely increased circulation. We go to the gym to increase circulation after strenuous exercise. We know that increased circulation is fantastic for the body. It means that everything is being fully supplied with all the blood it needs for optimum operation. The organs are pumping, the skin is flushing, the body is cleansing and processing.

- **Increases metabolism** If our organs and systems are being supplied with optimum levels of blood they can operate efficiently and perform their functions effectively. If our metabolism increases and improves, the rate at which the body processes foods and toxins, and burns energy, is also improved.

- **Increases pulse rate** When we get hot our pulse gets quicker and our heart pumps faster. A healthy heart can do this with no problem, but if there is heart disease this aspect of thermotherapy must be observed.

- **Increases cell metabolism** As well as organ metabolism becoming more efficient, the rate at which the body manufactures good chemicals such as hormones becomes more efficient or more balanced. This is a huge benefit of thermotherapy or hydrotherapy. Total balance can be achieved simply by balancing the body's exposure to heat and cold.

- **Increases lymph function** As the body is heated the blood pumps around the system and the tiny movements of the blood vessels increase the function of the lymph system – the body's waste-disposal system. This leads to increased internal cleansing and elimination.

- **Decreases the stimulus of the myoneural junction**
  Our muscles and nerves are constantly in communication with each other. We move our legs forwards when we think about walking; we sit up as soon as our brains hear the request; and we go to catch a falling object without any conscious thought – it happens automatically as our nerves yell at the muscles to lurch forwards. The application of heat slows that conversation down and everything goes into deep relaxation and reduced response times. When relaxed we move a lot more slowly. Heat relaxes the muscle response.

- **Reduces spacticity in the muscle**  The application of heat relaxes the muscles to the extent that we can do further work with the muscle fibres. We warm up before exercise to get flexibility. We get a massage and have our muscles warmed before the deep work occurs in order to relax the tension and melt away the tightness.

The application of heat allows our increased range in movement and reduces tension. The body becomes deeply relaxed and recovers, and repair takes place more efficiently. All these functions in isolation will increase and promote the body's ability to heal itself. Putting them all together for the 'short term' gives all these benefits almost immediately.

If only heat is repeatedly applied, it becomes 'long-term' application, and this becomes depressive on the circulatory system. Continued application of heat will result in the body taking up to a third of the blood away from the central organs and brain, to allow cooling; the body will feel very relaxed or tired. Long-term heat will feel uncomfortable and possibly claustrophobic.

Dizziness can be caused as blood is moved away from the brain when the body tries to cool itself. Heat applied over a long term will cause the body to try to cool down by pumping blood to the outer regions and skin, away from the core organs, to cool down and maintain optimum homeostasis, or balance of temperature.

## Cold

In contrast to heat, the short-term effect (two to five minutes) of cold on the body is much more refreshing and invigorating. We all know just how startling it is to have a cold shower. It is a total contrast to a warm, relaxing one! The short-term application of cold has the following beneficial effects.

*Application of cold:*

- **Causes vasoconstriction** In opposition to the relaxing of blood vessels that results when heat is applied, the application of cold will make the blood vessels constrict – a process called vasoconstriction. The narrowing of the blood vessels restricts the blood supply to areas and in effect pushes blood away from an area that was previously flooded with blood.

- **Produces an analgesic effect** The body releases a natural pain-relief substance (prostaglandin) into the muscle when cold is applied. This in turn reduces muscle-spindle spacticity and gives relief from the painful cramps of muscle tension. It also means in therapeutic terms that the muscles won't hurt as much if they are being worked or manipulated if the area has been cooled down in some way.

- **Provides a 'shock' effect of temperature change** When we experience the application of cold-water jets, cold showers, plunge pools, etc., one of the things that can be guaranteed is that a deep inhalation of breath will take place. We need to take a deep breath in order to catch our breath from the shock of the cold water. This deep breath makes us fully expand our lungs and therefore fully oxygenate our blood.

- **Inhibits the release of necrosin** This is a natural chemical that destroys tissue. If we damage a muscle this chemical continues to cause the damaged muscle to deteriorate. If you get the muscle cold as soon as you sustain any damage through injury, or perhaps through a hard workout or a deep-tissue massage, the damage will be limited because cold inhibits the release of this chemical and therefore muscle damage stops.

- **Reduces inflammation** When we are damaged or have over-used a muscle it is likely to become inflamed. This restricts movement around the area of damage for protection purposes, but it can also lead to a build-up of scar tissue that can eventually restrict movement in the long term. The application of cold will reduce inflammation by making sure that excess blood is pushed away from the area, keeping the swelling down and manageable.

The short-term application of cold is extremely beneficial, but over the long term it can lead to stagnation and a dangerous restriction of blood supply to an area.

When a combination of hot and cold application is delivered correctly, it is unparallelled in its therapeutic properties. Delivered incorrectly, however, it can be a mixture of hot and sweaty and cold and clammy, with no benefit. All it will do will be to check the body's ability to protect and survive, instead of rebuilding and regenerating. Hot and cold applied alternately will also help balance acidity and alkalinity (Ph) in the body.

The aim of LaStone Therapy is to cause a 'rollercoaster effect', or 'vascular gymnastics', using heat and cold alternately:

- Heat is applied
- Vasodilation
- Increases metabolism
- Increased pulse rate
- Increased circulation

- Increased cell metabolism
- Increased lymph function
- The body becomes deeply relaxed
- *Healing takes place more efficiently*
- The body eventually adjusts and homeostasis is reached.

THEN
- Cold is applied
- Immediate vasoconstriction
- Sharp intake of breath/oxygenation
- Analgesic effect
- Inhibits release of necrosin
- Reduction of inflammation
- Reduction of histamine
- The body pumps blood to the core organs to keep them warm and eventually adjusts so that homeostasis is reached.

THEN
- Heat is applied, and so on
- Cold is applied, and so on.

If heat and cold are applied continuously during the treatment there is a continuous process of vasoconstriction and vasodilation which results in increased flushing rates within the body and optimum healing. Heat and cold do more together than they can ever do apart.

Virtually everyone can benefit from a LaStone treatment. The chemical changes manifested in the body can be compared to a workout at the gym. They increase circulation, tone muscles, increase deeper breathing, and instill total relaxation, deep cleansing and processing of all organs, boosting the metabolic rate and systems and advancing immunity. There are hardly any conditions that would not benefit from this treatment. The ability to vary and thus tailor the treatment is simplicity itself. The ability to balance the client is profound.

If illness is imbalance, then LaStone Therapy is hugely beneficial in recovery or simply getting back to balance. The more variables the therapist has within any treatment, the more able they are to deliver the most appropriate treatment. In LaStone we have the variable of temperatures and time. Less heat for less time or less cold for less time; colder for longer or hotter for longer. All variables are possible. If the temperature of the human body is 37 degrees centigrade we have every temperature either side of this from freezing to 60 degrees centigrade. And we have all the time in a spectrum, from as short as 10 minutes to over an hour. We also have the variables of placement – what we put where and for how long. Excepting very few cases, anyone can benefit every time.

## The Further Beauty of this Treatment

Every treatment a therapist gives, both therapist and client receive. Temperature travels in every direction in the room and to the client and the therapist, so that the therapist's joints get the hot and cold thermotherapy, as well as the client's.

If we use essential oils both client and therapist will benefit. If we use crystals, the effect will benefit both, and if healing is used the energy will also be channelled through both.

Don't forget that one of the reasons why Spirit channelled this treatment to the person they did was because Mary Nelson was unconsciously and very consciously looking for some sort of solution to her problem of aching joints and damaged muscles. No matter how good we are ergonomically, and no matter how we try to apply pressure through correct posture and body weight, we still try to get to the best position to work a client's muscle even though we know it is not the best position for us as therapists. If you are reading this thinking the same, this is definitely the treatment for you.

The most common reason for attendance I am given by therapists on the training courses I host is that they are looking for a treatment they can practise that doesn't damage their joints or cause them pain during treatments.

This is a two way thing – total balance again.

## CHAPTER EIGHT

# Energy Work with LaStone Therapy

HAVING LOOKED AT the physical delivery of temperature and thermotherapeutic effects, we can now look at the energy and healing work within every LaStone treatment.

There are just a few steps that make a true LaStone treatment. These are as follows.

Start the treatment by:

- Respecting Breath.
- Respecting Mother Earth and Father Sky.
- The Spinal Layout – the stones the client lies on.
- The Opening Spiral – the auric field work.
- The Energy Connection – the placing of stones on the client's body addressing the chakra energy.

Continue with:

- Whatever form of bodywork or possibly no bodywork if the treatment is simply healing or energy work.

Finish with:

- The removal of the stones with breath work.
- The Closing Spiral – protecting your client.
- The Spinal Spiral – crystal work to stimulate the spinal flow.
- Smudging with sage, tapping of stones, or chiming of bells or bowls.

The honouring of the stones, the honouring of breath, the placement of stones and the energy work are what sets LaStone Therapy apart from all other treatments, stone or not. The respect for energy and the respect for nature is the key to this treatment.

## Working with the Breath – Our Own Life Force

LaStone Therapy honours breath, something we only notice when we are out of it, when we are short of it or when we don't have enough supply of it. If we don't take breaths we die.

I was first made aware of this in my adult life when I was on my trip to the US with my friend – the trip on which I discovered LaStone. We were asked to climb the telegraph pole, and were told to breathe steadily and gently. The first thing you do if you are scared is to hold your breath. This totally exacerbates the problem, making you dizzy and out of control. As I took my first step up the pole I was told to breathe. With every step I took I needed to concentrate on my breathing. This was the only thing that got me to the top – timing my breathing with my movements. As I reached the top I was asked to stand on the smallest disc possible. I could only do this if I took my breath deep down into my belly, my centre. As I did this, my centre balanced me and enabled me to take the next step. If I speeded up my breathing I got pannicky; if I slowed it down it was like a miracle. I was no longer quite so terrified – just because of my breathing.

If I was breathing properly, the pole was stable and I could hold my body firm. If I stopped breathing and began to let my mind take over with fear, the pole began to sway from side to side. Believe me, the best way to remember to breathe properly is to see how it calms a swaying twenty-five-foot-high telegraph pole!

A fellow guest managed to get to the top of the pole and the pole was swaying hugely from side to side. Breathe, we all said, softly but encouragingly. The reply was that she was breathing but the wind had picked up up there. We all knew from our recent experience that it was nothing to do with the wind. It was entirely due to the fact that she was not centring her breath and feeling grounded.

Breathing is the essence of life.

We take breathing for granted. We breathe all the time, and if we stop breathing for more than a few moments, we die. The last thing to leave our body as we pass away is our final breath. Our breath is an indication of how healthy we are, how calm we are, how centred we are and how we are feeling. We can use our breathing as a tool to enable us to do many things: to keep calm in a crises, to run a marathon, to dive to another world. The one thing for sure about our breath is that we take it totally and utterly for granted.

You may have read the section on how I personally discovered LaStone Therapy. It was on the same trip that I discovered how to use my breath to my advantage, to use it as a tool for survival and not just let it take control of me.

Honouring breath is a crucial part of LaStone Therapy.

Here is an exercise of breath with connection to Mother Earth and Father Sky, by the Reiki Master William Myers. The exercise is called 'Mother Earth and Breath'.

It has been said 'The truth will set you free.' Are we not the marriage, the blending of Mother Earth and Father Sky? A way to prove and claim our heritage is to breathe it. To share ten gentle, complete breaths first from Mother Earth, ground up, then Father

Sky, top down. You may begin with Father Sky first, as your heart guides you. Cherish their dance individually and then on the third set of breaths watch them join within you, creating body. This is a very accessible way to be family now, to share family every day, and to share our daily bread, our experiences with family. They miss us. As we receive a breath of life, watch it flow into ourselves, feet, legs, torso, and organs. As we give a breath, exhaling from our being, we can release our finished products for the service of others.

Every time a therapist places a stone on the body or removes it during a LaStone treatment, they honour breath.

You may be more aware of breathing when you are out of breath – for example when you are exercising. If your fitness instructor is doing their job properly, the term 'effort on the exhale' will ring a bell. Every stone is placed or connected with the body on the exhale, honouring the patterns of breath. Every stone is removed when the inward breath pushes the stone up and away from the client's body, as if to say 'Take this from me, I am done.'

The combination of the respect for breath and for Mother Earth is a unique element to body treatments and so to LaStone Therapy. Below is Mary's reminder of how we have forgotten about the things we did at play as children, and how, as adults, we have stopped respecting these important aspects of basic life.

I was shown this way of breath at a traditional Native American medicine conference. The medicine people shared that acknowledgement, that to honour daily breath ceremonies is most powerful. Breath is something we are all of the time. Can we savour it? We are creating a trillion new cells a day as body. Each cell is precise and precious. Can we feel it? As we make use of this simple breath, above and below and as one, we feel life's bittersweet embrace. If we can feel it, we can heat it. Let's call this 'Having a Near-life Experience'.

Something to think about. As humans we are drawn to hold Mother Earth next to us. While we were children we longed to get outside every day and play in the dirt and grass. We would lie on her body and feel the coolness of the grass, the warmth of the sand on a sunny beach; we even loved to walk in her waters or have rain fall on our faces. Children understand the need to be connected to Mother Earth and Father Sky; they seek them out daily, laughing and playing as though they had their best friend right beside them.

As a child you probably collected stones everywhere you went; most of us did or still do. You would see the beauty in a stone and want to hold the mystery of its energy near you, so in your pocket the stone would go. Once home you would add it to the pile of stones from days past and for a brief moment be able to recapture the heightened feelings of those other days of pure joy and excitement. What has happened to those stones we collected as a child, the memories of days past in the warmth of Father Sky and the beauty of Mother Earth all around us? We moved away from home, and where did they go? Outside to rejoin their clan, I hope, to resurface another day and bring joy to the next person who glances at their beauty.

As you begin your journey with the Stone Clan People, take a moment to recall some of these experience you had as a child. Recapture the feeling of being one with the world, knowing you are strong and can do anything. Do you remember that power you felt as a child when you got to the top of the hill? Breathe in the moment of pure joy once again and be one with Mother Earth and Father Sky. Touch the Earth and feel the warmth of the Sun on your body and breathe in pure joy, for you have found a lost friend.

Everywhere there is evidence of people needing to draw Mother Earth and Father Sky to them: we have pets in our homes, we plant flowers, we grow foods to eat. People carry and use stones for healing powers. We have paintings of the sky and the Sun within our homes. We love to sit and watch the Sun rise or set.

\*   \*   \*

Drawing in the power of the Sun rising or setting has been done for aeons, some people not fully understanding the need to be present at this daily event of Father Sky. We wear clothing from the creatures that move on this Earth. We've painted their like-nesses on our clothes and decorate our homes with them. Yet we as adults do not fully understand the power that can come from doing these things. These can be ways to honour Mother Earth and Father Sky if only we accept the powers within the symbols. Native Americans respected the messages that animal medicine can bring us and symbolise in our lives. Every animal has proper-ties we should know about, and we should use these messages to guide us in our daily lives.

Among the human populations on this Earth, many honour different clan families by using their likenesses for logos, such as a mascot for a team. Even without knowing it, they are using the energies of that clan to strengthen each one of them, and with any luck, the whole team. Think what power could be within each member of the team if they truly understood and accepted the power of the bear, for instance! From the book *Stone People Medi-cine* by Manny Twofeathers: '. . . Bear medicine gives you the ability to go as far as you need. To accomplish things that you might have thought were completely out of your reach. Yet at the same time, it brings you the wisdom to take only what you need, and go only as far as is necessary. It gives you the strength to conquer physical problems, and to overcome obstacles in your life. It can help you in your dreams, to recall them and find answers to your questions. Bear reminds you to be gentle with yourself, and others . . .'

At the end of this section there is a short summary of what some of the more popular animals represent in healing medicine. Take a look and see how Mother Earth gives us messages and help through the animals we encounter on a regular basis. You may already be thinking that a certain animal has been turning up more regularly in your life than usual. This is not just coincidence;

it is nature's way of trying to tell you something and help you. Mary says:

> Mother Earth and Father Sky give to us all that we need to survive. We only need to go and harvest our heart's desires and behold, our Mother and Father bring forth clothes to protect us, food to feed us, warmth and Sun to feed our bodies, and beauty to fill our eyes and spirit beyond anything we can create ourselves. The people on this planet need to take heed. If Mother Earth and Father Sky are to continue to give birth to even our simplest needs, we must begin to honour them, to give back what we have taken so freely. We have polluted his air, caused diseases to grow in her waters, ravished their four-legged clans, smothered so many different clan peoples. How then can we continue to take from the table they continue to spread before us? We cannot continue to do this without honouring them and all their clans. If we truly come from the clay of the Earth, then we are a part of our Mother Earth and all are brothers and sisters.
>
> To honour Mother Earth and Father Sky is to recognise their gifts, to see and feel the healing powers that are laid before us to use. One need only listen to hear the call of one of the clan families, as they reach out to the humans. Each member of a clan is willing to teach the human clan their powers, so that they can heal each other. Each clan family – the plants, animals, minerals and so on – wants to be of service to the humans. How are we repaying them for this endless service that all the clans have performed for aeons on our Mother Earth?
>
> Why are we gifted with such a high place in this chain of life, when we don't even honour our own role in the cycle of life? If we did act as true kings we would see to it that each clan was well provided for. We would hear their voices as they call to us to use them. We would know the power of our energies uniting. We would be worthy of a higher place in this universe.
>
> So I invite you to take a moment each day and go outside and breathe the strength of Mother Earth and Father Sky into your

body. Become one with the energy of the universe, giving thanks for what the day is about to offer you. Spread bird seed for the winged animals, feed the trees that shade your dwelling place and care for your Stone Clan family that now help you in your daily work.

# Animal Medicine

Animal medicine is the Native American way of empowering your life. It can enhance your belief system and it can become a belief system. Animals live on this Earth quite freely. They are wild, and they find ways to survive. When we domesticate them for our own pleasure and use they lose some of their independence but none of their 'animal instincts'. Pet cats will still bring in shrews, mice and birds, despite having a bowlful of food served to them on a regular basis. Horses at the riding stables will still shy away or kick out if you approach their blind spot. They are hunted in the wild and even though no one has ever left domesticated horses to the jaws of a wild animal, the survival instinct is in-built.

Each animal has properties we can learn from and use. Here is a brief summary of some of the more common animals.

## The Properties of Different Animals

| Animal | Medicine |
|--------|----------|
| Swan | Beauty and grace. Power from within. |
| Spider | New creations and creating new experiences. |
| Horse | Ability to travel and find freedom. Your own personal power. |
| Ant | Hard work will give you rewards. |
| Wolf | Guarding and protecting. Loyalty. |
| Owl | Truth and vision. |

| Animal | Medicine |
| --- | --- |
| Dolphin | Breath and life. Joy. |
| Bat | Facing your fear. Seeing through everything to get to the truth. |
| Deer | Caring, compassion and gentleness. |
| Bear | Power. Physical and inner strength. |
| Dog | Loyalty. |
| Squirrel | Preparation; being industrious and prepared for any eventuality. |
| Coyote | Having fun, lightening up, not being so serious. |
| Whale | Creativity. |
| Eagle | Getting things in perspective; taking the bigger view to sort things out. |
| Snake | Change, rebirth and wisdom. Magic and enchantment. |
| Butterfly | Transformation and change. |
| Fox | Cunning. Imagination and interpretation. |
| Crow | Magic and change. Secrecy. |
| Cat | Independence and mystery. |

If any of these animals has been appearing more often or even for the first time in your life they may just be trying to get through to you. Animal medicine is empowering and will keep you young forever. Animals do not work with your age; they work with your being.

# Spinal Layout, Auric Field Work and Chakras

Clients are placed on stones, have energy work to open them out for deep relaxation and healing, and have stones placed on them

– all in the first few moments of the treatment. In less than ten minutes your experience will be deep and profound and like nothing you have ever experienced before. Then you will still have sixty minutes to go – total balance and total bliss.

We will now look at each of several aspects of the treatment in much more detail to find out exactly why they are so important. The use of basalt and marble in LaStone Therapy is unique. The combination of energy work and the stones makes the treatment profoundly unique. Each of these parts of the treatment is valid, effective and deep, put together to become an experience. This is what makes LaStone Therapy the most exciting therapy available today. I will argue that point until the cows retire and come home to spend their twilight years in rest and relaxation. The stones are important and the treatment couldn't happen without them. Breath work is crucial and we ignore this to huge detriment in the treatment. The energy work is important and the treatment is also incomplete without it. This is what sets LaStone Therapy apart from other stone work available today.

In LaStone Therapy we believe that the subtle energy of the stones works together with the chakras and the aura, so there is no formal chakra opening and closing. What we do, however, is proper stone placement. This means that together with honouring breath and energy we place hot, cold or neutral stones on the chakras, while incorporating a sequence of moves to connect them all together and open out the client into their auric field or potential.

This is called the Opening Spiral pattern – and upon completion of the body work or stone work we carry out the Closing Spiral pattern. The whole process optimises the client's ability to open up to receive the treatment and removes barriers from the therapist, enabling them to work deeper and on a more profound level for the client. I sometimes compare this to spring cleaning. If you simply wash the surfaces and tidy the items around you things look good for a while but this doesn't last for long – all it needs is a spill or the messing up of a tidy pile for the work to be undone. If, however, you actually open the cupboards wide and tidy deep into the backs of them, removing everything that has passed its sell by date; if you put everything in its proper home and not just in a tidy pile, the effects will last a lot longer, continuing long after the work.

A treatment without the opening work is like a quick wash and brush-up, while a treatment with the opening energy work is a total remodelling. They both cost the same, but which would you rather experience?

## The Spinal Layout

The very first thing we give to our clients in a treatment is the Spinal Layout. After taking a case history we can decide on the correct application of temperature, but the true first contact with the stones is when you roll the client back onto those spinal stones. Each stone is placed in a way that will be most effective for the client at that time, and to stimulate or relax the nerves along the spine and send balancing messages to the brain and central nervous system. The temperature immediately begins work on manipulating those tired and over-worked back muscles while talking to the rest of the body.

## The auric field

The concept of the aura and chakra system was developed in ancient Far Eastern cultures. These cultures believed that there was a dynamic energy field surrounding the physical body. There is no 'proof' as such of the layers of light or spiritual energy, but the experiences of therapists and energy workers alike show that there is a great and deep belief in their existence and their effectiveness.

In fact, there has been extensive research carried out by many experts into the biomagnetic field (aura) of every living organism, and there seems to be no question of the existence of electrical fields around the body.

Dr Valerie V. Hunt, a neurophysiologist and psychologist at UCLA, developed instruments that could demonstrate high frequencies emitted from people's bodies. These frequencies could also correlate with auric colours reported by clairvoyants working with the project. She verified that there are two electrical systems in the body. The first is the system aligned to the electrical current of the nervous system and brain, while the second is a continual electromagnetic radiation coming from our atoms, which allows an energetic exchange between the individual body and its environment. Therefore, anything that consists of atoms, which is everything, has an energy field or aura.

Many cultures talk of the Universal Life Force, sometimes called Prana, Ki or Chi or Qi. Individuals can draw energy from this pool to remain balanced and healthy in mind, body and spirit. They can also draw energy specifically through the chakras, or wheels, positioned in key areas of the body. These areas can be described as individual spinning wheels of energy within the whole subtle energy system, or aura.

If a person is in total balance and health then everything is spinning at the correct rate for that specific individual. If anything is out of balance then either the excess or the deficiency can be worked on through the chakras and auric fields until balance is attained.

We can say that the aura is a subtle light that surrounds absolutely every structure. This also offers protection. In healing worlds the colour of this light can be seen, and the density determines how active or spiritually developed the structure is.

We can think of the aura as the ripples in a pond; if the pond is clear and we throw something in it, the ripples flow freely outwards and around the object in perfect harmony. If there is anything in the way, such as a twig or weed, the ripples stop at the point where they touch the obstruction. Doing energy work with the chakras and the auric field will remove the blockage and allow the ripples to continue undisturbed. Before we go on to look at the chakras and their corresponding fields we can also mention here that in most treatments, therapists will be familiar with seven main chakras. After Mary studied Brugh Joy's work she was happy to see that her 'opening spiral' had included contact in twelve places – more than the normal allocation of chakras. Brugh Joy helped her by explaining that he had identified many, many more chakras than have been used previously in most therapies. As a result, we can add ankles, knees, splenic, higher heart and transpersonal points to our chakra description, and therefore to the opening spiral pattern.

### The opening of the auric fields

We don't just aim to open up the auric fields in a random process. Each layer looks different and represents different aspect of a structure, person or object. Also, each layer of the aura has a relationship with a specific chakra (*see opposite*). The main chakras directly correlate to the main layers of the auric field. Chakra one opens and relates to the first layer of the field, chakra two relates to the second, chakra three to the third and so on.

Each layer has its own colour, luminescence or radiance. Indeed, there is a form of light photography that can show the colours and energy surrounding the body. Kirlian Photography can reveal the colours that are dominant in the aura at one particular time. The therapist or individual can then work accordingly on boosting or decreasing energies until the individual is in balance.

## Energy Connection and Proper Stone Placement on the Body

In LaStone Therapy, once we have opened a client's auric fields, or their potential, or if you like to think of it as just relaxing and smudging their edges so we have full access, we place stones on their body. We place them on the chakra points using energy connection. This ritual connects the body with Mother Earth, the stones and the temperature. We place specifically and synchronise the placement with breath. This completes the beginning of the LaStone treatment.

## The Seven Main Chakras

| Names and characteristics of the main chakras | Corresponding layers of aura and colour |
| --- | --- |
| **Root**<br>Physical being and physical needs, success in physical and material matters. | Physical and material health.<br>Red. |
| **Sacral**<br>Emotions and feelings, sexuality, giving and receiving, trust in relationships. | Creation.<br>Orange. |
| **Solar Plexus**<br>Personal power, self and mental thought, letting go of ego. | Emotion.<br>Yellow. |
| **Heart**<br>Humanity, love for fellow man, personal love and relationships, balance. | Humanity, forgiveness.<br>Green. |
| **Throat**<br>Communication, power of the spoken word, self-expression. | Communication.<br>Blue. |
| **Third Eye**<br>Celestial love, intuition, imagination and wisdom, higher thought. | Intuition.<br>Indigo. |
| **Crown**<br>The bringing together of spiritual and physical life, total spirituality, wisdom and the higher self. | Spirituality.<br>Violet or White. |

# Crystal Work and Energy from Crystals

During a LaStone Therapy treatment there is the opportunity to introduce many forms of crystal work. Two techniques were incorporated into the original LaStone Therapy treatment which are encouraged for every treatment. These are the Spinal Spiral using a piece of flourite or a flourite wand, and the use of labradorite for cleansing and neutralising the stones during the hard work they do.

## The Spinal Spiral

We have looked at the Opening and Closing Spirals in the section on energy work, and now we can introduce another stroke and crystal that could even be a whole treatment on its own.

The Spinal Spiral is a sequence that addresses every vertebra of the spine, from the top of the neck to the tail bone. It is extremely relaxing and is used to ground and centre the client after the potential 'roller coaster' of temperature and mind, body and spirit work that they have just received. The work involves both sides of the spine and stimulates the nerve path on either side. The right-hand side of the body represents Spirit or the past, and the left rebirth or the future. Again, you can see that it is in total balance; the work involves the left and right, the spiritual and the physical, and the sequence grounds after the client has travelled.

This stroke can be done with your finger, but we now tend to use a crystal called flourite, or Chinese flourite. This crystal has many properties, but the reasons we choose to use it for this part of LaStone is because:

- **Spiritually**, it stimulates a free spirit. It makes us aware if people are trying to control us and allows us to ignore these outside influences. Flourite makes us creative and inventive.

- **Emotionally**, flourite makes us aware of supressed feelings. It allows us to see them gradually, so that they do not cause an outburst of uncontrolled emotion. Flourite opens us up to our subconscious. It has a balancing and stabilising effect on our emotions, gives us self-confidence and clears any confusion.
- **Mentally**, flourite dissolves blockages, fixed ideas, stubbornness, narrow mindedness and small thinking. It helps us to process thoughts usefully and works as a learning aid to cross think, broaden horizons and associate. Flourite stimulates rapid absorption of information and quick thinking.
- **Physically**, flourite stimulates regeneration of the skin, mucous membrane and lungs. It strengthens the teeth and bones, and helps with postural problems. Flourite aids mobility and improves stiffness in the joints – so it is especially good for arthritis. The activity of the nervous system is encouraged and psychosomatic allergies are alleviated by flourite.

Flourite is best used directly on the body. It is ideal for use in the Spinal Spiral.

## The Five Elements in LaStone Therapy

Each of the five elements is used in a LaStone Therapy treatment. They are earth, fire, metal, wood and water. This observes the Chinese five element beliefs.

- The earth element is the most important in this treatment and it is involved in the use of the stones, the marble and the crystals.
- The fire element is the electricity to heat the stones.
- The metal element is the heater used.
- The wood element is the sage, the wooden spoon and the fabrics and towels (fabric comes from plants, which are part of the wood element).

- The water element is the water the stones are heated in and the ice we use to cool the marble.

Yet again, this treatment demonstrates total balance of all aspects. As Mary Nelson says so simply in this letter to students, the combination of this respect for different energetic beliefs, different forms of healing, breath and energy work, only adds to the layers of this fabulous therapy.

> It is my deepest feeling that when you bring the stones into massage, you must honour the breath of the client with this union. As you begin to use the Opening Spiral in each treatment, you will see that the client becomes less resistant to this joining of the stones to their bodies.
>
> In doing the Opening Spiral you assist the client's auric fields to open and expand, allowing movement of energy within the field. By touching the chakras in this order you bring fuller expression of the field into the client's awareness. The touching of the chakras is not intended to open or change the flow of the chakras themselves. The touching of the chakra in combination with the Opening Spiral is like using a doorknob on a door, a way to make the field wider and more open to receive information. As you join the client's body at the point of each chakra, use their breath. Allow your touch to join their body with each exhalation, as the chest is growing smaller, and sinking in, as if to say, 'Here I have made a place for your hand to rest.'
>
> As you complete the Opening Spiral and begin the Energy Connection, maintain the flow of energy by having one hand on the client at all times. If you take both hands off the client at the same time, you break the flow of the energy that you began at the Opening Spiral. It is so important to understand this next step. The body is electrical, and your touch is connecting electrical impulses from joint to joint and chakra to chakra. If you remove both hands, even for a split second, you will disconnect the flow and the moment will be lost.

Holding the ankles, with the client's breath begin the Energy Connection. To join the body with the breath, watch the chest as it moves up and down. Some people will breathe more slowly than others, and some may breathe rapidly. If your client seems to be breathing at a fast pace, ask them to take a few slow/deep breaths. Maintain the hold on the ankles (lightly) and let them bring their breath into rhythm with this connection.

Move one hand at a time from joint to joint and then chakra to chakra. Join the hand to the body as the client exhales and leave the body as he or she inhales. Use this method of joining the body with either your hands or the stones. Allow the body to accept the stone or your hand as it makes room for you and the stone. Be willing to leave the body when the chest becomes large (inhalation) as though you were being pushed off, saying 'Now it is time to leave and I will help you move away.'

Do you see how important it is to bring and release energy in this way, with the breath of life that fuels your client's body?

Whether you are doing the Opening Spiral, the Energy Connection or the Closing Spiral, or joining or removing the stones to and from the body, you must honour the client's and the stones' breath of life. The rhythm of breath with the hand and stone placement will bring your client into a fuller understanding of their connection with Mother Earth, Father Sky and their own spiritual being. For me this is what will make or break your treatment with the stones.

Having respect for breath, the Earth, the Sun and the Moon, the animals, and everything nature has to offer is crucially important for our survival. I have said this earlier in this book, but we need to remember that we can only live successfully if we respect the fact that we live off things this planet creates – water, wood, metal, fabrics, foods, animals. If we lose respect and take things a little too much for granted, we will fail. If we think we are in charge, we are sadly mistaken. Nature is definitely driving the car and we are simply passengers.

Our resources need to be respected.

## So What Do the Stones Think?

Mary wanted to know what the stones thought of her work and if they approved of it, and whether she had heard them correctly. To this end she met with a person called Valerie Sorrells, who is a medium. Together, through discussion and receiving treatments from Mary, Valerie was able to receive feedback from the stones.

One of my clients introduced me to Valerie Sorrells in the summer of 1994. Valerie channels for people, so I asked her if she could channel for the stones. I wanted to know where I could get more of their kind, for they are very rare in the Tucson area. I was also interested to know if the stones liked the way that I was using them and whether they were willing to share anything more. Valerie agreed, and I let her take the first stone I pick up to use in massage. It was very hard for me to let that stone out of my sight, but I trusted that she would take care of the stone and that the stone would be returned to me. Valerie returned my stone and gifted me the channelled information that she had received from the Ancient Ones. [The Ancient Ones are the stones on this planet. See Further Reading, *page 131*, for Jamie Sams and Twylah Nitsch's book, *Other Council Fires Were Here Before Ours*.] I then gifted her a massage with the stones. I usually only take an hour to do a massage. This night more than ninety minutes passed before I began to close the treatment. Valerie and I both went out of body during this treatment. Since then, whenever I work on Valerie, I can plan on travelling to dream places with visions of the spirit world. I only have a few clients who are open enough for both of us to travel and dream while I work on them. If you are blessed with a client such as this, give thanks to all that exist, for this is a most beautiful blessing and one to be thankful for.

## The message from Valerie Sorrells from the Stones

My message comes to you, Mary, down through the ages. The Spirit of my Ancestors existed at the dawning of this planet's existence. We have existed here for millennia, serving to strengthen the energies on this planet.

We have been brought forth at this time after aeons of preparation. Our form has been perfected for the methods which you would work with us. Through the action of the running waters our edges have been smoothed to a state which is pleasing to the human being's physical form.

We have much to teach the children of this age. Our hardiness speaks to you of endurance and strength. We who were created through action of explosive flames, mirror for you your creation in light and from light. Our firmness speaks to you of the solidity of your human frame at the present time, but our inner energies remind you that you are children of light.

The frequencies contained within us can aid humans in reprogramming their memories and accessing their awareness of who they are as children of light. We arise on the planet at this time in our perfect form for human touch and examination.

As such we can be touched and caressed lovingly by humans, and they shall receive our energies. We can be carried in the clothing as well. We can be rubbed on the body by a separate individual or the person to be massaged can rub themselves, and still utilise our energies.

Our energies penetrate the muscles, tendons and ligaments, and move deeply into the bones, accessing deep genetic and ingrained memories. Our energies are deep and penetrating. They are slow and warming. You have enhanced our energies by your use of heat and water in our preparation for use with human beings. We are fond of our connection with the fiery light and liquid waters.

We would encourage you to continue our use in your practice. I would encourage the use of fifty-two stones. Continue your current patterns, but add patterns of use under and over the arms and legs, as these long bones are quite receptive to our energies. Also focus on areas of the skull, as our energies can penetrate and vibrate through the skull to brain tissue and glandular tissue in the brain area, further stimulating recall and enlightenment in the human form.

Our use over the energy centres is of a deep, penetrating nature. We serve not so much to open the centres (although we may), as to balance and ground the centres once they have been opened by other methods. Our use in opening the centres is limited due to our lower frequency; higher frequencies are needed to open stubbornly closed centres (Oh, how stubborn humans can be!).

We would ask you to consider using us with cooling methods as well. There is a balance to our nature, and it may be of use in situations where cooling is in order. Recall how we love the frigid cold of a running river! You may experiment with cooling us in iced water or through other methods that enable cooling. We would be used in cool form over isolated areas where cooling is indicated, for example over burns or over areas that are over-active with energy. Heaven knows, humans would certainly throw us off themselves and crush us if there were too many of us on them at once! We have no desire to unnecessarily irritate anyone!

You wish to know where to find more of us. We are scattered all over this Earth in various pockets of concentration. Many of us are now buried in icy places you would know as arctic areas, where we will surface at later times. Yet those of my immediate family can be found in this country [the United States], and I would suggest you search in the cities of Oregon, namely Portland.

It is so wonderful to communicate with you like this through this channel. Know that you, too, can receive information from us directly anytime you wish, as we have a special connection which has formed over the aeons. Your Spirit is deeply connected with ours, as yours is with this channel, and this channel is with us. We are all working together for the healing of the planet and all of creation. We love you dearly, Mary, and support you with our loving energies. We appreciate your work and dedication towards surfacing our energies on the planet. We close now, with love in our hearts and wishes of peace and happiness for you.

*The Ancient Ones*

You may find it difficult to see how the stones can give messages about how they wish to be used, but you probably don't find it too difficult to believe in intuition. No one questions a mother's intuition if something is wrong with her child – even if the child is many miles away. Intuition – as I have recently learnt – is tuition from within. So anything that comes to mind, that you hear within yourself or that you think about or imagine, can be described as intuition.

You may be happier thinking that the message from the stones is purely intuition, but whatever the source, the thoughts are valid and came from somewhere.

When you start to include stones in your life you will begin to know what is meant by this. It may even be time for you to open yourself up to your own inner teachings – your very own IN-TUITION.

Mary Nelson trusts her own intuition, and we encourage every LaStone therapist and every client to develop and trust theirs. If a thought comes to mind it is probably your own inner teacher – your 'in' tuition. Next time this happens, go with it and see where it takes you. Listen to your heart and act on the information it gives you. From Mary:

Intuition: we all have it. Some of us listen and respond to our inner voice, our Spirit, as if it were a friend giving us advice. We must tap into our own inner teacher and begin to trust the messages that come through to us from the spirit world daily. Each of us receives messages on an on-going basis; we just choose not to listen. We are either too busy in our daily lives, or we think 'I can do that later', or 'Do I know you? You seem so familiar to me', or 'It feels as though I have been here before'. We have all felt and said these things, passing them off as coincidence or *déjà vu*, not realising that our Spirit travels ahead of us, and that it knows the future and remembers our past lives.

On a very special level our soul knows and remembers all there is to know of the entire universe. We, on a conscious level, just choose not to remember, not to pay attention, or feel that if we start to buy into these day/night dreams, someone might think we are crazy and lock us up. The challenge to believe the thoughts ourselves is at times most difficult. That is why we spend a life-time trying to tap into our inner teachers, not even realising we are connected to the collective consciousness. It can be such a lonely life – looking for an outside teacher and not realising our Spirit is our truest form of knowing.

Begin to listen to your inner teacher, and allow the voice to guide you in the simplest parts of your everyday life. Then you will begin to hear messages from the spirit world, and at that time you will know the truth that governs all the universe, that all is unfolding as it should.

We agreed to experience these events in our lives with certain individuals. The growth we are passing through is at this moment travelling at the most divine speed. We need not feel we are behind, for when you are on a spiritual path you are always at the beginning. You have begun the awakening process that never ends.

This type of listening is what takes place when you let yourself hear the stones give you directions. A voice speaks to you from deep within your soul. Trust that it is divine inspiration and not a part of your thinking mind that you have no control over the process. Give in to the soft voice that is pointing the way to a higher state of healing. Using the stones with massage, energy and light work, you will be able to enhance all bodywork treatments beyond anything you have previously experienced.

One of the most direct ways that I receive messages from the stones is by laying them out on the massage table, lying down on top of them, and placing the rest of the stones on top of me. I go into a dream-like state within seconds after getting the stones just where I want them, or, I should say, just where they want to be. During this time of rest I receive information about the use of the stones by sensing how it would feel if they were used in this way or that way. Then I try out the new ways on the next client, and always ask for feedback on how they responded to the new technique. My clients love to try new ways of using the stones, so they are willing to let me continue to add more of Mother Earth's energy into the massage by way of the stones. I also receive messages from the stones while working on someone or when I receive LaStone Therapy from one of my students.

To help you understand and recognise these messages, here are some examples from my experiences. I was working on a regular client who had just gone through leg surgery for the second time, when I kept getting a picture in my mind of a chisel and hammer. I have learned not to question or even to judge, but just to use the stones in the way that they are directing me to use them. So I chose two stones and began to work with them on the leg until they lost some of their heat. While holding one stone over the area of tension, I began gently to tap that stone with the other stone, maintaining a rhythm of music that radiated into the body from the stones. When I asked the client how it felt, the reply was, 'Great, I felt the vibration go deep into my leg, into the bone. I like it.' This soft tapping of the stones over a tight area sends waves of vibration deeper into the soft tissue, and with the warmth of the stones, the muscles give way to the tension, while the bones receive the soft waves of vibration. The stones love to talk, so experiment with the music that comes from them when you bring two of them together.

The way I received the message about the stones is quite funny. I was massaging a man from Russia who spoke very little English, and I speak no Russian. While working on him, I kept hearing 'Use the stones between his toes.' I thought, sure, now how do I explain that move? The voice kept after me until I took the two eye stones and placed them between the first two toes of both feet. For the first time in the massage the man spoke: 'That is wonderful. I love putting things between my toes.' I breathed a sigh of relief and thanked my spirit guide for this new technique. And yes, the next day I was out harvesting toe stones. I now use eight toe stones on everyone.

Listen to the stones as they speak to you through your inner spirit, and allow the thoughts and images that come into your consciousness to guide you along a path of awakening, both for your clients and yourself. Know that the stones that came from Mother Earth are here to help you and your clients to reach deeper levels of understanding of the path you are on, and that healing stones pave a road before us that reaches not only into the past, but travels into the future for insights on healing and releasing blocked memories and pain. Allow yourself to hear these messages, and use them as they call to you.

Keeping an open mind as a LaStone therapist is clearly what makes the best, and the most imaginative and innovative treatment. Every time you receive a treatment as a client, and every time a therapist gives a treatment, it should be a totally individual therapy. Even when they honour the essence of the treatment, the places you go to and the effect it has on you will be unique but totally appropriate for you at that point in time. You will achieve balance – a great place to be.

## CHAPTER NINE

# Practising LaStone Therapy

THE WORD 'THERAPY' is important in this treatment, as I have discussed. To that end we can see that there are many ways to receive the treatment. It doesn't always have to be in the form of massage directly onto the skin.

## Oil-free Massage

An oil-free massage using LaStone Therapy can be done by incorporating one or more forms of energy work into the treatment, as well as applying some massage strokes, such as trigger-point work, piezoelectric effect, holding, vibration, rocking the stones, and toning. A total full-body treatment can be carried out without a client needing to remove any clothing. Remember that the temperature travels through the fabric of our clothing.

This form of treatment may be required if the client has any of the contraindications for Swedish massage, or if it is their first massage and they are a bit wary of taking off their clothing.

It is still possible to lay on the stones, to make the Spiral Opening, to have stones placed on the body and to have pressure-point work done slowly and methodically through the clothing. Fresh stones can be used and then tucked alongside the client so that the temperature surrounds them.

There really isn't a reason to not have some form of LaStone work – clothed or unclothed, lying down or sitting up, relaxed or invigorated, in isolation or as an integral part of another therapy – to start or end the day.

## Home Visits

It is possible to have a mobile LaStone Therapy treatment, involving a visit by a therapist to your own home. There is a bit more work involved not only for the therapist but also for the client who is requesting a home visit. A large amount of equipment needs to be transported to the client's home, but it is entirely possible to do a mobile treatment. This is how Mary goes about her home visits.

I load all my massage items into a large carpet bag I made from upholstery material. The stones are placed in the roaster just as they normally would be, without the water. This way of packing gives me just three items that I need to bring into the client's home: the carpet bag, the roaster and the massage table. At the time you set the appointment ask the client if they are willing to have one or two gallons of hot water on their cooker ready for you when you get there. This will save you twenty to thirty minutes of heating time. Also ask for a small table to set the stones on. The first thing you set up when arriving at the home is the roaster and the stones. Always, even in your office, place a towel under the roaster to absorb any water that may drip off as you are pulling stones out. You'll also need a towel next to the roaster to set the stones on, to remove a bit of the hot water before you take them over to the massage table and the client. If you take dripping wet stones to the massage table it will not be pleasant for the client to lie in a puddle of water, not to mention the fact that water will be spilled on the floor. Once the table and stones are all set up, pour the hot water over the stones in the roaster and set it at its normal setting to give you a temperature of about 50 to 55 degrees centigrade. Once the stones are heating, set up the massage table and oils as needed, and by that time, five minutes or so, the stones will be ready. You can be set up in less than ten minutes and be ready to go to work if the client heats the water for you in advance.

If you are prepared to help your therapist, you should be able to have a wonderful experience in your own home.

## Other Types of Therapy with LaStone

As mentioned before, LaStone Therapy doesn't have to be normal massage. There are many courses available for the therapist to take which will both broaden their horizon and extend your treatment choice.

If you are a client, whatever your treatment rest assured that your therapist has undergone thorough training in their chosen subject, and that in turn their instructor has been tested to even greater lengths before being able to call themselves an instructor. At LaStone we expect the body of knowledge and experience our instructors have to be far, far greater than any therapist can use in any course.

## The Training Your Therapist Has Taken

Each LaStone therapist must already be a qualified therapist and have a minimum of 500 hours practice time – hands on bodies to you and me! Most have considerably more. In fact, the more experienced the therapist, the easier they will find the transition from 'hand work' to 'stone work'.

LaStone is therefore termed a 'post-graduate course'. We do not train non-therapists. Your therapist has trained for three and a half days in their chosen LaStone course. The training is intensive. During the training the therapist discovers the theory of LaStone and its origins – in fact, almost everything in this book is taught as basic knowledge for a therapist. The LaStone training does not dictate exactly everything that must be done in every treatment, but it does aim to open the mind of the therapist and to enhance their current skills with the use of the stones. Aspects of the treatment like the energy work and connection work should be respected during any genuine treatment, and the combination of the use of hot and cold stones is imperative. A treatment without cold is not a LaStone treatment.

The therapist is asked to carry out nine 'give aways' that they can use as practice sessions on friends and family in order to make sure that the treatment is ready and practised before beginning to charge their clients. LaStone is a very difficult therapy to learn but once mastered it is the most amazing therapy and definitely worth the work.

There are several LaStone courses a therapist can consider.

## Original LaStone treatment

Original Body may be the first and only course that Mary Nelson currently teaches but there are many ways to experience LaStone Therapy. It is, however, likely that the treatment you will have first will be a full-body Original LaStone.

Once you have tried this amazing experience, you could go on to search out therapists who are qualified in many other LaStone techniques. Indeed, you can check what level your therapist practises. A LaStone therapist has completed one training course in any of the techniques – usually Original Body.

## Advanced LaStone therapist

An advanced therapist has taken four different courses in LaStone Therapy of those listed below. This shows their ability to adapt the treatment to their current therapy qualifications on several levels.

## Master LaStone therapist

A Master LaStone Therapist is qualified in over seven of the therapies listed below. Master LaStone therapists are fairly rare, but if you ever do meet one you will be in extremely skilful company.

### Beyond Basic

Completion of this course will mean that your therapist has taken further study to expand their knowledge on the basic principles from Original Body. The alternating temperatures are really examined and deep work on specific muscle groups is a big consideratuon. Working muscle groups in order for tension, blockage and emotional release to move through and out of the body is considered.

### Deep-tissue Course

This course covers the use of hot and cold stones for deep-tissue work. In this class the therapist learns how to use the stones for deep-tissue work, such as trigger-point work, positional release and cross-fibre friction, as well as side positions for deeper work. Information is given about different body types, sports activities, job-related injuries and postural difficulties. Incorporating the stones in deep-tissue work enables clients to heal and at the same time takes them to a level of relaxation they have never been to before with deep-tissue work.

We all know that this can be painful but it isn't the case with stones involved. The use of frozen stones for injuries as well as alternating hot and cold stones for tissue repair and stress reduction allows relaxation during deep manipulation. In turn this promotes healing, and for days after the work gives relief from chronic and/or acute problems a client may have been trying to live with or get used to.

## 'Simply' training courses

The 'Simply' group of treatments is designed to introduce the therapist, spa or salon to the beauty of the stones in shortened and slightly modified treatments. The treatments do stand alone but they also demonstrate how valuable the range of skills is to have.

### Simply Stones

This course enables the spa groups to introduce stone work into a fifty-minute treatment. The art of alternating temperatures is used in the shortened treatment to allow the spa schedule of one-hour turnaround to operate unhindered. The experience will bring the guest back time and time again as they see how even in just a short time they can feel the penetrating benefits of the temperatures. In this course we teach techniques for applying heated and chilled stones to the body, and cover contraindications and considerations for this 'mini' full-body treatment.

Students also learn how to clean the stones, and how to care for all the supplies necessary to bring this little oasis of calm and tranquility into a shortened fifty-minute spa treatment. Proper body mechanics in relationship to the stones are also taught; these help to protect the hands and wrists of therapists from the additional strain of being overworked when they have daily 'back to back' treatment schedules.

## Simply Faces

Therapists learn stone and thermotherapy techniques that they can integrate into their current mini facial or full facial. Placement of the stones, and their care and cleansing, is incorporated into this two-day course. Swedish strokes are taught using heated and chilled stones on the face and neck, arms, hands, feet and lower legs.

## Simply Beauty

Simply Beauty is a natural extension or simple introduction to the Original LaStone Therapy course. It is designed for the successful beauty therapist looking to upgrade their existing skills. Introducing the stones into your daily treatment menu will transform the results for your clients in just a few simple but effective steps.

Simply Beauty covers LaStone waxing, manicure, pedicure, facials, extractions and much more. No massage techniques are taught on this course, but the many ways you can use the application of thermotherapy through the stones will become invaluable in your current treatments. By adding LaStone to your therapy you will be starting out on a relationship that can work for all your modalities, massage, aromatherapy, reflexology, remedial work and healing.

## Stone Chi Therapy

Stone Chi Therapy is a four-day journey into the application of hot basalt and cold marble stones with chakras and meridians. The traditional Chinese medicine theories of internal heat, cold, damp, dry and wind are examined in relation to working with the perfect yin and yang balance of the stones. You look at deep energy Tsubo (pressure work) and resolving internal conditions. This course will appeal to anyone who is trained in shiatsu, acupressure or Chinese medicine, and would like to add the powerful dimension of Earth energies to their practice, integrating hot and cold stone work with the complex meridian work that they are already doing.

## Stone Facials for the Soul

This course involves learning the use of hot and cold stones for aesthetic work. You learn the principles and benefits behind thermotherapy – how to use hot and cold stones in your facials, and the proper placement of the stones on your body. The stones will bring a deeper state of relaxation to your clients. By the end of the course, you will have an understanding of the stones in relation to the ever-growing search for true body, mind and soul philosophies in your work.

## Stone Soul Connection

The use of hot and cold stones in reflexology work brings new levels of relaxation to your clients' feet. In this course you learn how to substitute a warm or cold stone for your tired thumbs. In combination with specially blended oils for LaStone Therapy, your clients will begin the process of healing through the soles of their feet. You learn the secrets behind LaStone Therapy theory and philosophies, and thermotherapy principles, and bring the energy of Mother Earth into your reflexology treatments.

## Not Just Polished Stones

You learn how to incorporate Mother Earth energies into your manicures and pedicures, and bring the body, mind and soul connection into the glamour of salon life. You will be able to aid your clients to relaxation through the use of warm stones, and help to eliminate sore hands and feet with the use of cold stones. Bring the energies of Mother Earth into the glitter of painted nails and see both the inner and the outer beauty that your clients walk away with.

## The training the instructors undergo

Becoming a LaStone Therapy instructor involves a very extensive programme. Our therapists need to be skilled in instruction and therapy – one without the other is not acceptable.

Here is a copy of an e-mail response from Mary Nelson to a prospective instructor.

The following are guidelines. Over the past nine years we have trained 27 individuals to teach the LaStone Therapy techniques; we have revamped the requirements many times. Our goal is to produce the highest level of instructors this world has in geo-thermotherapy, LaStone techniques and energy work modalities. We are most honoured when someone is willing to take the time and effort to study at this level of intensity.

These are my criteria:

- Once a year in the spring the Board of Directors gathers and votes on all applications for the TCP, the Teacher's Certification Programme. There is no promise made that anyone being accepted into the programme will be able to complete all requirements. This is on an individual basis.
- The therapist has taken at least one workshop with LaStone Therapy.
- The therapist has practised the LaStone Therapy techniques for a period of one full year. We feel strongly about this, for how can one teach others a technique if one does not have practical knowledge of what they are teaching? One needs to be able to answer multiple questions in regard to contraindications and client considerations and needs.
- The therapist has been a body worker for at least five years. The therapist has taught something, anything, for at least one year.

- The therapist has no less then 1,000 hours in body therapy school and or continuing educational hours.
- The therapist studies with our senior instructors. This usually means six or more workshops as a teacher-in-training. The time-frame for this is from six months to two years. I have seen some individuals complete the requirements in as little as six months, and we have had a few that took two years. This is very individual, and dependent on how one learns and the time that can be committed to learning.
- The time frame for completion of the TCP is around 180 hours.
- Once you are an instructor we hold yearly up-grades for all instructors here in Tucson. The Skill Enhancement workshops for the instructors are mandatory in order to remain an instructor of LaStone Therapy. These Skill Enhancement workshops are a time for up-grading your teaching skills, bonding with all the instructors from around the world, and sharing your teaching experiences with one another.
- The annual affiliation fees for instructorship will be discussed when you are wanting to take on this responsibility.
- As well as the hefty requirements for training, the potential instructor is required to show the ability to host classes, to have sufficient equipment to hold a class and to make sure the students' needs are met at all stages.

This may seem very hard and you may wonder why there isn't a straightforward course that one can follow to become an instructor. The answer lies in the need for LaStone to maintain the extremely high standards that are attributed to the Original Stone therapy. LaStone was the first manifestation of stone work on the body in modern times and as such sets the standards that all others follow.

There are barriers to entry and these are high standards, huge efficiency and an extremely effective, physical and spiritual, deeply profound treatment. Once a therapist has demonstrated their ability to fulfil all these criteria, they may be considered to hold the title instructor.

# Other Expressions of Stone Therapies

As with anything that is good, there will be groups bringing out similar versions that use the same techniques, and try to improve them or emulate them. This is extremely flattering and it is now possible to see many different types of stone therapy on the market.

LaStone Therapy was and is the Original Stone therapy in the modern day. However, as mentioned previously, there is absolutely nothing new about the treatment. It is simply Mary Nelson's channelled message and her experience, experimentation and wisdom that have given us the LaStone treatment we know today.

The fact that there are now many types of stone therapy does give therapists a problem. Are they as good/better/worse than LaStone Therapy? Is there anyone in competition in my area? I don't want to tread on anyone's toes ...

My advice is to chill. If your concern as a therapist is that you may lose business to other companies or therapists, then just make sure you practise, and honour the stones and yourself, and then see what manifests. If you stay small and secret so that you don't show your skills and don't give anything away, then – according to the laws of Karma – you will get nothing in return (Karma is the Sanskrit for come-back). Conversely, if you put out skill, good intentions and healing – the results will be terrific.

Mary Nelson is often asked the following questions. What are you going to do? Have you protected your rights? Have you got a lawyer? Have you made sure you own the treatment? Why don't you sue? This is her response.

In 1995, when Bonnie and Elka [two students on one of Mary's first LaStone courses] began to teach the use of hot stones in massage, Tomi and I were devastated. Patricia and Teresa were able to help us see a higher story, and yet that did not ease the pain of betrayal and thievery that we felt was being inflicted upon us.

As the years passed, more and more former students and outsiders began to copy the teachings of the stones and to water down the foundation of what was gifted to me through prayer and chan-nelling. All instructors and honourable students were seeing this as treachery and a dishonest means in which to make a buck. How dare someone steal from the teachings of LaStone Therapy or read an article and have the audacity to copy Mary's work! During those dark and shadowy years we were all blinded by the gift that Spirit offered each of us and the hunger that humans have for their Earth Mother. We continued to refer to these thieves as *Copy Cats* and turned our backs on the question of why they felt the need to copy the magic of Mother Earth and her Stone People.

In 1999 we grew up a little and started to understand the process of the *Copy Cats* and therefore began to refer to them as *Followers*. We convinced ourselves that we understood why others took it upon themselves to recreate what we felt we had mastered in the art of Stone Therapy.

Now in this new millennium I understand why others have been and will forever be drawn to the magic of the stones and the deep connection one feels with Mother Earth as stones are glided across the body. It is my hope that in the next few sentences I can assist you all in finding within your own soul an acceptance of the *Other Expressions of Stone Therapies* just as I have come to find comfort and support in this process.

From the beginning of time humans have used stones to facili-tate healing within the body. We have brought this knowledge into Swedish massage, deep-tissue massage, Shiatsu, reflexology and all types of body therapy. We who are the stewards of the stones' magic are the fore-founders of this new and ancient form of body healing. LaStone Therapy woke up the massage world to an ancient art of healing. In this millennium we were the first to bring alternating temperatures to the body via stones in a treat-ment.

Each of the *Other Expressions* offers us a challenge to be the best we can be; to up-grade and do research on what it is that we are teaching; to offer new and expanded forms of therapies to the body in conjunction with hot and cold stones; to explore the use of different types of stone in alternating temperatures, from the smallest dense basalt to the largest quartz crystal one can place on or around the body. It is our agreement with the stones, with Mother Earth and with our own souls that we should find ways in which to awaken humanity to the magic of the Stone People.

According to this agreement, it is our duty to allow others the same privilege of exploration. How can any one of us say to another human being that they cannot hear the voice of Spirit and be enlightened and guided by the force of the universe? Surely there are souls working with the stones that have no conscious connection with Spirit or Mother Earth. Search your own soul. Do you really feel that Mother Earth or the Great Mystery would play a part in a treatment if they were not willing to be a part of the experience? Thus some of the *Other Expressions* will be connected to Spirit and the Stone People and some will not. The ones that are I send blessings to and encouragement to seek out more. The ones that work with the stones for money and profit only, I send blessings to and encouragement to seek out more. As the founder of LaStone Therapy I ask all that are in our community to do the same: open your hearts and minds to the *Other Expressions,* and see them as healthy competition and a means by which you will strive to be the best LaStone instructor you can be.

Let us look at other types of competition out there in the world. How many department stores are there in your local area? How many car dealers are there out there all claiming to be the best or the first at what they are selling? Each of them believes they are the best or the first; each of them does research on what the market wants or what is selling. They are all surviving and even thriving. They all support one another in odd ways – one may offer what another does not, and research constantly reveals new and better ways in which to build and market their products. The consumer finds interest in the method used and the information provided to them to make a choice. There is no difference in the *Other Expressions* of stone work. We are the *First Expression* of hot and cold stone work in modern times. If we stay committed as a group we will be the *Last One Therapy, LaStone Therapy.*

I thank all of you who have ears and hearts to hear what I am expressing in this story. It is my prayer for all of you that any and all competition will be welcomed into your energy field and not rebutted. Grow and develop a higher understanding of your commitment to the stewardship of the Stones' Magic.

With love and blessings,

Mary Nelson

Founder of LaStone Therapy

# Index

# About LaStone Courses and Treatments

The only legal documentation we issue to therapists is designed to protect the clients. Those that choose to, pay us for treatments. Their monetary exchange for our LaStone skills is greatly appreciated and we don't wish to restrict this flow. What we do hope to restrict is anyone using the stones when they do not fully understand the implications of the treatment on every level. The training to become a LaStone therapist allows the client to receive the best treatment for them at that point in time – a treatment to take them forwards and to progress.

You are only able to carry out a LaStone treatment if you are a qualified LaStone therapist taught by a qualified LaStone instructor. It is that simple and it is all we ask.

## Developments for the future

Who knows where LaStone will take any of us? All we do know is that LaStone Incorporated is dedicated to increasing its knowledge and understanding of the power of this treatment. We are sure we have merely scratched the surface. Each time we have time, each time we have funds, we use them to develop the knowledge and increase the learning. Each instructor remains in contact with the skills-enhancement courses. Even if they simply grow from exchange and experience, this is still passed on to therapists as they train. LaStone Therapy is a moving target and we hope never to pin it down. We have put it out there and we eagerly await to see what comes back.

## Contact details

All LaStone therapists are invited to subscribe to the LaStone Therapy web site. To find someone in your area please check under your country and area.

### International web address
www.lastonetherapy.com

### UK contact and training
LaStone Therapy Ltd
London, England

E-mail
Jane@lastonetherapy.com

Contact numbers for course information in the UK
Debbie Thomas
0208 291 5890

### USA and international contact
LaStone Therapy Inc
Tucson, Arizona

E-mail
info@lastonetherapy.com